the geriatric aide

Gail D. Kuhn
March 3, 1978

the geriatric aide

Jane Henry Stolten, R.N.

Little, Brown and Company, Boston

Published December 1973

Copyright © 1973 by Little, Brown and Company (Inc.)

First Edition

Third Printing

Library of Congress catalog card No. 73-2030

ISBN 0-316-81741-4

The photographs on the cover, title page, and pages 1, 25, and 259 are by Michael G. Reed, courtesy of The Day Hospital, The Burke Rehabilitation Center, White Plains, New York.

Printed in the United States of America

This book was designed and written especially for you so that you can learn to understand the needs of older patients, to meet their needs in the best ways and to love your work and the old people you will meet as a geriatric aide. I stress *love*. Old people respond to love or the lack of it above all other things.

Scientists have found that plants react to the interest and loving concern of those who tend them. Plants thrive and blossom if they are spoken to, sung to, or otherwise acknowledged, admired, and emotionally nourished. Plants shrink from attendants who do not value them; they wither and die under indifferent care. If plants respond so strongly to human love, surely humans do.

Old people have much to offer if allowed to express it. Each patient possesses a lifetime's individual wealth of knowledge and experience. You can share in this wealth if, while tending to their bodily needs, you consider each patient as a person. Communicate with that person in every way that you can; through smiles, touches, soft, reassuring words, warm feelings, sharing, joking, listening. Listening is very important. Really listen when the person speaks. Listen and respond to what is said. By so doing you reach the speaker's feelings of trust, appreciation, and affection; the person blooms and reveals his or her unique beauty. Such bloomings are the sweetest of all nursing rewards. Because there is ample time for personal relationships to develop, geriatric nursing offers more opportunities for these rewards than do other areas of nursing practice.

If you love your patients, you will love your work. If you love your work, you will work well. If you work well, you will be happy, content, and fulfilled. If you are happy, content, and fulfilled, you will give off good vibrations that make others happy. If you make others happy, they will love you.

You will learn best if you understand how to use your book. Take a few minutes to look through it to find the following:

Table of Contents

Just before the text is a Table of Contents. This is a listing by chapters of all the general subjects you will study. After each subject is the number of the page on which that subject is discussed. Read through the listing once to become familiar with the subjects. Thereafter refer to the Table of Contents whenever you need to locate information about a general subject.

Study Guide

At the start of most chapters you will find a Study Guide of questions. Read all the questions for one lesson before you begin that lesson. Reread the questions and look for the answers in the text. Say each question and the right answer aloud. Try the questions again after you have studied all the answers. Check your answers by referring to the lesson. Try the questions again after a week. Ask a friend to help you. Get him or her to ask the questions one at a time. Answer each question aloud. If you are unsure of any answer, look it up again in the text.

Cross-References

While reading about a subject, you may come across a reference to another part of the book. For example: (*See* "Collecting Specimens" in Chap. 14.). This is a *cross-reference* and means that more information about the subject can be found under the topic referred to.

Sample Examinations

On pages 323–324, you will find some Sample Examinations, made up of *yes and no* questions and *multiple choice* questions. These are the kinds of questions you may be asked on an examination. Practice for an exam by writing the answers to these questions in your book. Use a pencil. Check your answers with those that appear on the answer page. If you are not satisfied with the answers that you wrote, erase them and do the entire test again. Recheck the answers.

Index

At the back of your book is an index. This is an alphabetical listing of the subjects in the book and the page on which reference to each subject can be found. If, for example, you want to find out about wheelchairs, you would turn to the section with *w* letters and then look for words having a second letter *h* and so on until you locate the entire word. For wheelchairs you will find:

Wheelchair(s), 86, 103–106
    accessories for, 104
    activities in, 80
    care of, 104–105
    care of amputee in, 294
    cut-out seatboard use in, 184,
        186–187
    general duties to patient in,
        105–106
    manipulation of, 103, 115
    moving forward in, 105
    restraints for, 22, 51
    sizes of, 104
    transfer of helpless patient to,
        165–166
    transfer of patient from bed to,
        162, 164
    transfer to straight chair from,
        164–165
    types of, 103–104

The page numbers directly after the term direct you to where the subject is discussed throughout the book. The terms indented below the main heading direct you to *specific* discussions. For example, if you are just interested in a wheelchair for a helpless patient, the index entry directs you to pages 165–166. Correct use of the index will save you time.

Student Work Record

The final page of your book is a Student Work Record. This is a record of your overall progress during aide training. You and your teachers can tell by a glance at this record sheet what you have completed and what you must do.

You will hear lectures during your training period. However, the first lecture that you attend may not be Lecture Number 1. Your teacher will announce the number of a lecture before it is given. At each lecture period, circle the announced number.

Your teacher will inform you of the program number and the demonstration subjects for that program. Write the subjects, exactly as given, beside the number listing for the correct program.

The list of demonstration subjects is followed by four columns of blanks. The blanks will be filled in by your teacher who will write the date that you first observe a demonstration and, later, the date that you have practiced it. And, if you practice the demonstration again, the teacher will record that date also. When satisfied with your performance, the teacher will write his or her initials in the last column to show approval of that demonstration.

A completed Student Work Record should indicate to you, and to your teacher, that you are ready to take a final examination on work covered by lectures, demonstrations, and related reading assignments.

I hope that you will enjoy your book and use it not only to study during your training but to refresh your memory during the many years you plan to work as a geriatric aide.

With all best wishes,

Jane Henry Stolten, R.N.

TO THE INSTRUCTOR

The 1971 White House Conference on Aging examined a decade of public and private efforts to meet the needs of elderly citizens. One conference consideration was the quality of nursing care being delivered to the nation's geriatric patients.

In this respect, the conference found the nation as a whole to be wanting. Although the elements of excellent geriatric nursing care were known and were being put into practice in some superior systems of nursing-care delivery, national distribution of this knowledge was inadequate to serve the majority of geriatric patients who were receiving less-than-adequate specific care.

The conference recommended that specific education in geriatric nursing care be given to all nursing personnel involved in caring for the elderly; it cited a particular need for this education to extend to aides, since they had frequent, close contacts with patients.

The Geriatric Aide responds to that need. It offers the elements of geriatric nursing care as taught to and practiced by aides in some of the health systems that were upheld as models by the 1961 and 1971 White House Conferences on Aging. It presents these elements in clear, easy-to-read instructions and uses proved educational methods that appeal to and encourage students. Because a picture of total nursing care is desirable, the book is not limited only to specific geriatric methods but includes relevant basic nursing-care procedures with emphasis on adapting these to the geriatric patient.

The text is intended for use in programs designed for the in-service training and upgrading of aides in those hospitals, nursing homes, day-care centers, and home-care systems that service some or only geriatric patients. It is suitable for use in four progressive courses in the upgrading process.

Program 1 should introduce general concepts of geriatric and rehabilitation nursing care and should review basic nursing procedures in the light of these concepts.

Program 2 should expand on geriatric and rehabilitation theory and teach specific techniques related to the theory.

Program 3 should teach procedures that require conditions of judgment, work experience, skill, and confidence. (*Example:* condom drainage assembly.)

Program 4 should concentrate on special health conditions in geriatric patients and on the specific care for each condition. (*Examples:* diabetes, chronic brain syndrome, cerebral vascular accident.)

Programs 1, 2, and 3 should include ten or more one-hour lecture periods and ten or more two-hour demonstration and return demonstration periods.

A lecture period may include a film or other teaching device, a talk by a guest speaker or the instructor, an oral or written quiz, a homework assignment of reading from the text, and a question-and-answer time. Lectures should stress theory and complement or stress text material. As many as 30 students may attend a lecture.

A demonstration period should present specific nursing care procedures in a practice environment and stress developing skills and confidence. Each student should be allowed to proceed at his own rate. A ratio of no more than ten students to one instructor is desirable.

On the last page of the book is a Student Work Record sheet which allows a student to record his own attendance and progress at lectures and demonstration periods. If an instructor numbers a lecture series to correspond with the numbers across the top of the work record sheet, the instructor can inform the class of the lecture number at the start of a lecture period, and each student can circle the appropriate number on his work record. Topics, selected by the instructor as suitable for demonstrations, may be written in the left-hand column of the demonstration record. The instructor should consider a student's work record at the close of every demonstration period and initial any work completed during the period. Two or three simple procedures may be completed in a single period; a more difficult procedure may require one or more entire periods.

A work-time differential of six months to one year, between Programs 1 and 2, is advisable. A work-time differential of one or more years between Programs 1 and 3 is advisable. Program 3 should be offered only to those with outstanding abilities.

Program 4 may be offered concurrently or between courses one and two. Association of each topic with a patient known to the students is highly desirable.

It is hoped that this book will help in raising the standards of nursing-care delivery to geriatric patients and add to the work enjoyment of students.

J. H. S.

ACKNOWLEDGMENTS

I wish to acknowledge and thank the following sources of help and material:

- The Rusk Institute of Physical Medicine and Rehabilitation, New York
- The Jewish Home for the Aged, New York
- Kingsbridge House, New York
- Mary Manning Walsh Home, New York
- Goldwater Memorial Hospital, New York
- Loeb Center, Montefiore Hospital, New York
- Visiting Nurse Service, New York
- St. Joseph's Manor, Trumbull, Conn.
- The Burke Rehabilitation Center, White Plains, N.Y.
- H.E.W. Day Hospital Research Project at the Burke Rehabilitation Center, White Plains, N.Y.
- Birch Wathen School, New York
- The American Foundation for the Blind
- The Salvation Army
- The 1971 White House Conference on Aging
- Reports of the Congressional Special Committee on Aging
- Health, Education, and Welfare Publications:
  - "Step into Action"
  - "Services Available for Nursing Care of the Sick at Home"
  - "Strike Back at Stroke"
  - "Handle With Care"
  - "Elementary Rehabilitation Nursing Care"
  - "Protective Services Project for Older Adults"
- Journals of the American Geriatric Society
- Reports of the National Old People's Welfare Council (England)
- Army Medical Department Handbook of Basic Nursing
- "Basic Nursing Ward Procedure Manual – Rehabilitation Monograph" – New York University Medical Center

J. H. S.

Part I. On Being a Geriatric Aide

Part II. Meeting Your Geriatric Patient's Needs

14. YOUR GERIATRIC PATIENT NEEDS BOWEL AND BLADDER CONTROL   219

15. YOUR GERIATRIC PATIENT NEEDS MEDICATION AND INHALATION THERAPY   249

Part III. Special Conditions of Your Geriatric Patient

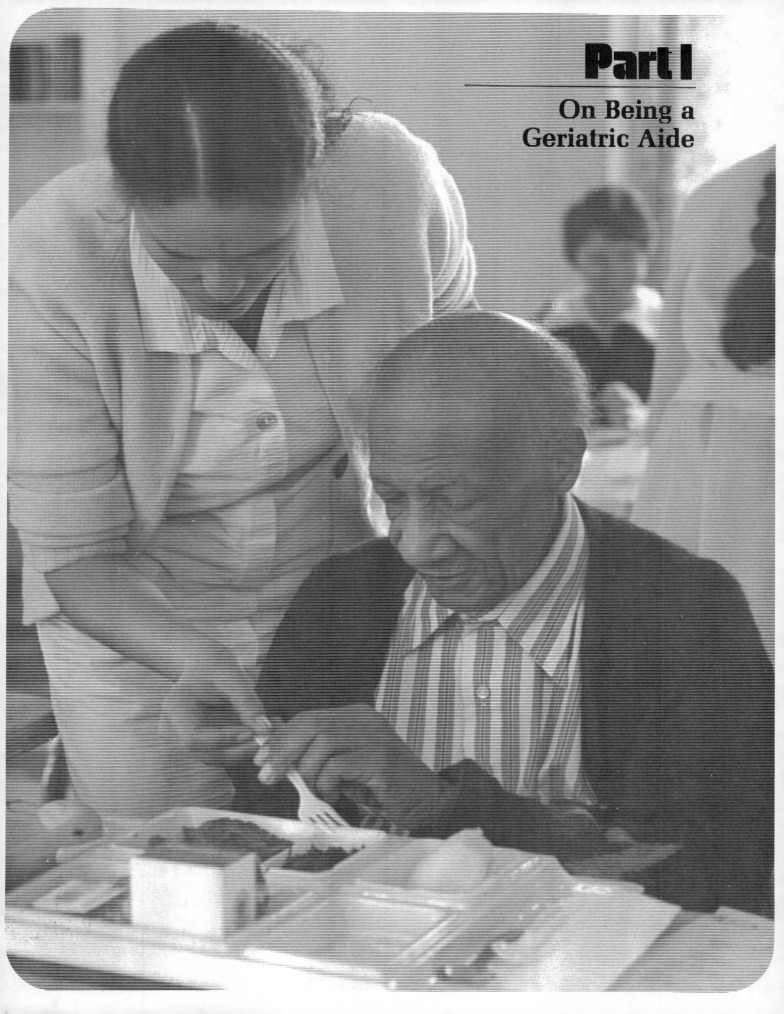

Part I
On Being a Geriatric Aide

THE QUALITIES OF A GERIATRIC AIDE

STUDY GUIDE

Working as a Geriatric Aide

What is geriatrics?

What is a geriatric aide?

What special qualities should one have to work in nursing?

What other qualities should a geriatric aide possess?

How should a geriatric aide dress and act?

What can you do about the way older people react to smells, noise, and movements?

What kind of check should you give yourself before going on duty?

What six responsibilities do you have as an employee?

Speaking on the Telephone

How should you answer a telephone when on duty?

What five things should you write down when taking a message?

What should you do before making a telephone call while on duty?

The Nurses in Charge and You

What responsibilities does the charge nurse have?

When should you report to the charge nurse?

What can you expect from the charge nurse?

How can you check yourself before going off duty?

The Doctor and You

What might a doctor expect from you in a nursing home? At home with a patient?

When taking a patient to a doctor, what should you also take?

By what titles are doctors who specialize in the care of the aged called?

What should you do before telephoning a doctor?

What information should you give when you have reached the doctor, his office, or his answering service?

What should you do with any information you receive over the telephone from the doctor, his office nurse, or the answering service?

The Geriatric Patient and You

What three things must you consider when you care for any patient?

What factors cause differences in each person?

What is aging?

How does aging affect the geriatric patient?

What are the medical goals of geriatric care?

What emotional stresses affect the health of the geriatric patient?

How might a geriatric patient express his fears?

How can you help a geriatric patient feel at home in a nursing home?

Why and how do family members occasionally distress a patient and nursing home staff?

How do you learn to deal with family behavior?

GERIATRICS is the study of the diseases and care of old people.
  Geriatric care is a special form of nursing that meets the needs of the elderly.
  A geriatric aide is one who gives care to older people.

CAN YOU BE A GERIATRIC AIDE?

The fact that you are reading this page shows that you are interested in health work.

Only certain people are interested in the sick and needy. In fact, throughout history people with these interests have been so unusual that they have always gained the respect and admiration of their fellowmen.

Interest is not enough, however. You need to have some special qualities that will help you to learn. How many of the qualities listed here do you think you have?

  Good manners
  Tact
  Neat appearance and working habits
  Honesty and dependability
  Sincerity and an unselfish nature
  Calm nature
  Willingness to accept directions
  Cooperativeness
  Competence to do a task exactly
  The ability to learn
  The ability to observe
  The ability to adjust to many changes

A geriatric aide also needs other qualities besides those just named. Do you have these additional qualities?

Patience
Cheerful nature
The ability to work at a slower pace
A genuine liking for older people

Geriatric aide training not only helps you to develop these qualities, but also teaches you the nursing arts that can make you aware of the individual needs of each patient, lessen the distress of the patient and his family, and save the patient and you from unnecessary wastes of time, effort, and supplies. These are the arts that can give you that deep satisfaction unique to the field of health care.

Do you think you could learn these things?

Maybe you know an aide who is one of the many thousands now working in geriatric nursing homes, private homes, and hospitals throughout the country. Ask him or her. Any aide can tell you of the many students who doubted themselves. Some thought they did not have enough education or were too old to learn. Most of those who were interested enough to try were surprised because they did well. Determination and dedicated teachers helped them through even the most difficult challenges.

You can be a geriatric aide if you try.

GERIATRIC AIDES ARE NEEDED

The United States has an estimated 20 million people over the age of 65. This large number of older people is a result of a better standard of living and better prevention and treatment of disease. Because of continuing advances in medical knowledge and the worldwide population explosion, the number of people who will live to old age is expected to increase.

These facts have prompted government on federal, state, and local levels to examine the needs of the aging and to seek ways to meet them. Increased Social Security benefits, tax exemptions, medicare, nursing homes, day care centers, and nursing services for the aged within their own homes are some of the many results of the investigations of the needs of the aging.

The increase in the number of geriatric nursing homes and day care centers and the provision of home nursing care services for geriatric patients have opened a large and expanding field of employment for geriatric aides.

MEN AS GERIATRIC AIDES

There is a demand for men to work as geriatric aides. Since World War II, men serving as medical corpsmen have proved they possess all the qualities desirable for good nursing care. They have some additional assets too. For the most part, they are stronger, more mechanically minded, and less prone to show emotional stress than are women. There are many areas of geriatric care in which these additional assets are preferred. Men make excellent health aides and are needed to fill many positions.

WHAT GERIATRIC AIDE STUDIES CAN MEAN FOR YOU

The demand for men and women to work as geriatric aides has resulted in salaries and benefits favorable to these employees. Good work is needed and is rewarded with job security. Good work as an aide ensures a good standard of living.

YOUR DRESS AND GENERAL BEHAVIOR

The ways in which you dress and act as a geriatric aide are very important. Clothes and actions that are admired elsewhere may be offensive here.

All health workers are expected to be conservative in their dress and behavior. Personal cleanliness is essential.

General Rules

Take a bath and change your underwear daily.

Use a deodorant.

Brush your teeth and use a mouthwash.

Shampoo your hair often, keep it trimmed, and wear it arranged neatly off your shoulders.

Trim your nails short. Do not wear colored fingernail polish.

Do not wear jewelry except for a wedding ring and a wristwatch with a second hand.

Take good care of your uniforms. They should be comfortably loose and of moderate length. Keep them spotless, mended, and with all buttons attached. Always have a spare uniform ready. Some nursing homes furnish aide uniforms.

Take good care of your shoes. Invest in comfortable, low-heeled, well-fitting shoes with nonskid soles. Keep them clean and polished. Repair run-down heels.

Take good care of your duty stockings or socks. Keep them clean and free of holes, ugly runs, and wrinkles.

Invest in a plain, dark blue or black sweater. Keep it for duty use only.

Wear your uniform with pride. Express your pride in good posture, good manners, and good relationships with your patients and fellow workers. Be formal, not familiar. Call everyone by his right title. (*Example:* Dr. Jones, Mrs. Smith.)

Remember that older people react to smells. Don't wear strong perfume or cologne. Don't smoke in uniform. Don't eat foods such as garlic just before going on duty.

Remember that older people react to noise. Try to walk, speak, and work as quietly as possible. Don't bang, drop, or drag things.

Remember that older people are aware of movements. Don't, for example, bump, jar, or lean against occupied beds, wheelchairs, and walkers.

Organize your work to prevent unnecessary steps. Locate all the equipment you may need to use so that you are prepared to get it at a moment's notice. Check equipment before using it. Check, clean, and return every piece of equipment to its place after use.

Ask for help if you need it. Never be afraid to ask questions about anything that you do not understand. Asking questions or asking for help may prevent you from making a mistake. Make every effort to avoid mistakes, but *do* report it to your charge nurse if you make one. It could mean a difference of life or death for your patient.

The first rule in nursing is that the patient is always considered before anything or anyone else. Observe this rule. Listen to your patient when you are on duty and do your talking at home. Keep your personal life and problems to yourself; don't worry your patient with them. Work when on duty and enjoy yourself on your free time.

Dressing and behaving in these ways dignifies you and your work and helps you to get the most benefit for your efforts. You increase your knowledge, your satisfaction, your ability, and your chances for promotion.

Before going on duty you should stand in uniform before a full-length mirror and check your appearance and personal equipment, such as a watch and pen.

ASSUMING YOUR RESPONSIBILITIES AS AN EMPLOYEE

Certain obligations are implied in any agreement that is made to work. This is as true for a geriatric aide as for a person working in industry, government, or elsewhere. It is true regardless of whether you work for a hospital, nursing home, registry, doctor, or private family. It is understood that you will do the following:

Report on duty, in uniform, a few minutes before time for you to start work.

Try never to be late. If you are detained unavoidably, notify your employer before the time that you are expected to report on duty.

Notify your employer in advance if you cannot work on a day that you are scheduled to work. Then he can get someone else to work in your place.

Don't discuss the personal affairs of your employer at work or away from work. This includes information about the nature of the illness of a patient. You should talk about the patient, his illness, and his treatment only with the doctor, the charge nurse, or other medical workers who must know.

Do your best to build and maintain a good reputation for yourself and your employer.

Give at least two weeks' notice when you intend to leave employment. This means the employer has a chance to look for someone to replace you.

If you do fulfill your requirements and do good work, you will soon find yourself appreciated. Then in the event that you leave a job, you will have good references.

Many employers give new aides sheets of rules and regulations, which should be thoroughly studied before starting work.

SAMPLE SHEET
RULES FOR A GERIATRIC AIDE

We welcome you as part of our nursing team and wish to inform you of the following:
1. *YOU WILL START* as a_____ on _____ on _____ .
   You will begin at _____ and will work until_____.
2. *ALL NURSING AIDES ARE REQUIRED TO:*
   a. Wear white uniforms.
   b. Wear beige or white stockings.
   c. Wear closed, low, rubber-heeled, comfortable white shoes.
   d. Refrain from wearing gaudy jewelry and makeup. You may wear a wristwatch and wedding band.
   e. Keep hair neat and well-groomed.
3. *ALL NURSING AIDES ARE REQUIRED* to work a five-day week, including Saturday and Sunday. The nursing office assigns days off. You will be given a weekend off according to the rotating schedule.
4. *TIME CARDS* are used for recording time. You will be instructed on the use of these cards.
5. *LOCKERS WILL BE ISSUED* for your personal use. Because of a lack of lockers, you may be required to share one. A combination lock is provided. Please keep your locker locked at all times. You are not permitted to bring pocketbooks or coats to the floors.
6. *ASSIGNMENTS* are made by the nursing office. You may be sent to any department that needs help. Assignments are not permanent and you may be rotated to other departments periodically. You may be asked to work overtime when necessary.

Expected on Duty	Call Prior To
7:30 A.M.	7:00 A.M.
3:30 P.M.	12:00 P.M.
12:00 A.M.	3:00 P.M.

7. Report to your department administrator immediately if you have an accident or if you become ill on duty. It is essential that an accident report be filled out before you leave the floor.

8. *YOU ARE PAID BY CHECK* every two weeks on a Wednesday. Your starting date will determine the amount you receive for each payroll period. You are not paid for the week you receive your check. You are paid for the prior two-week period.

9. *ALL NEW EMPLOYEES* are on a probationary period for the first six months of employment. If you are involved in any of the following actions, it will result in immediate discharge:

    a. Deliberate violation of instructions on the nursing unit.
    b. Failure to perform duties according to procedure book.
    c. Unexcused lateness or absenteeism.
    d. Performing duties outside of the realm of your training.
    e. Failure to conform to recommendations found in the Policy Manual of the home.

10. *NO TELEPHONE CALLS* will be received directly by employees while on duty. Necessary messages will be taken and given to you.

11. *UPON SATISFACTORY COMPLETION OF YOUR PROBATIONARY PERIOD,* you will become a permanent employee and will be entitled to sick leave and vacation credit according to the home policies. The amount you are entitled to will be explained to you by the person in charge of personnel.

12. *FOR GENERAL NURSING INFORMATION* and other bulletins you should be aware of and read the BULLETIN BOARD located by the time clock.

If you have any questions, or problems related to your work, please bring them to the attention of the Nursing Office.

SPEAKING ON THE TELEPHONE

An important part of any health training is to learn to save time in as many ways as possible. One recognized way of saving time is to answer the telephone in a brief, but informative, way. Speak slowly and clearly.

Learn not to say "hello" when you answer, but rather to give the name of the place where you are situated at that moment, and then to give your own title and name.

Example: "Division Two. Aide, Mrs. T. Smith speaking."
                or
    "Mr. George Jones's residence. His Attendant, Mr. Parker, speaking."

If it is necessary to take a message, write it down.

Get all of the following information: the date and time, the name of the person who is to receive the message, the name of the person who is calling, and the message. Then sign your title and your name, or your initials.

Example: Dec. 6, 1970. 10:45 A.M.
        For Aide, Mr. G. Barker
        The nursing office called. Miss Greene would like to see you this afternoon at
           3:00 P.M. J.S.

Either deliver the message to the person for whom it is intended or give it to the ward clerk to deliver. In the absence of the clerk, give the message to the nurse in charge.

Be just as careful when you place a call to any person or service connected with the medical profession. Before you call, know exactly what you need to relate. As soon as you are connected, identify yourself and your location. Then give the reason for your call.

Example: You must contact the laundry because no towels were sent with the other clean linen:
        The laundry answers, "Laundry, Clerk Johnson speaking."
        You reply, "Division Two. Aide, Mrs. T. Smith calling. No towels were delivered with
           the clean laundry today. They were listed on the requisition slip. I have the floor
           copy sheet in my hand."

Because the telephone is an essential part of any institution's functioning, a duty phone must never be used for personal calls. Personnel, patients, and visitors should use the pay telephones that are located for their convenience in every hospital or nursing facility.

THE NURSE IN CHARGE AND YOU

The charge nurse has many responsibilities. She is responsible for the safety and comfort of every patient under her care. She is responsible for seeing that each patient has the care ordered by his doctor. She is responsible for seeing that the floor has sufficient workers at all times. She must know where every patient assigned to her care will be at all times. It is very important, therefore, that you know what you should expect from the charge nurse and what the charge nurse expects from you.

The charge nurse expects you to report to her at the following times:

1. When you begin your tour of duty.
2. Before you leave the floor for any reason (and you must tell the reason). (*Example:* "I am leaving now to take Mr. Jones to x-ray.")
3. When you return to the floor from anywhere. (*Example:* "I am back from taking Mr. Jones to x-ray. He is still there. X-ray will call when he is ready to return.")
4. When you have finished any work she has assigned to you.
5. When you notice any abnormal condition in a patient or a visitor.
6. When you discover that a piece of equipment is out of order.
7. After you have given any treatments that must be charted.
8. Before you report off duty at the end of your tour.

You can expect the charge nurse to do the following things:

She will give you your daily assignment and explain what is to be done for each patient under your care. Carry a small pad and pencil with you. As the charge nurse reports on each patient assigned to you, write the name, room number, and bed number of that patient. Then list the special care.

Example: Mrs. C. Smith   Rm. 456   Bed C
        complete bed bath
        turn every two hours
        pressure sore — intensive skin care — lambskin
        side rails up

Mr. T. Black   Rm. 430   (private)
out of bed
shower
have ready for x-ray by 10:00 A.M.

As you go about your work, make a check after every completed task. Then you always know what work is finished and what is yet to be done.

The charge nurse makes out the duty and days-off schedule. You must tell her well in advance of any special days off that you want. She will try to arrange them. It is not always possible, however, to have off the days that you request.

The charge nurse tells you when to take your lunch period and when to go for coffee breaks. These times are arranged around patients' needs, so all members of the staff must take turns.

Before reporting off duty, check your assignment sheet and each of your patients. Be sure that you have done everything.

SAMPLE DAY ROUTINE FOR AIDES IN A GERIATRIC FACILITY

7:00 A.M.–8:00 A.M.

Sign in.

Report in full uniform to the charge nurse.

Listen to the report on the patient by the charge nurse.

Take written notes on your daily assignment.

Check the rooms of all patients assigned to you. Speak to each patient. Question them about unusual problems. Take care of immediate needs. Check the daily schedule of each patient and see that each is prepared for and on time for appointments.

Answer signal lights promptly.

Give help with baths, showers, and other morning care to your assigned patients.

Help with dressing, oral hygiene, shaving, and grooming.

Collect and test urine specimens of diabetic patients.

Check urinary drainage equipment. Change drainage from bed bags to leg bags on out-of-bed patients, when needed.

Help patients with braces, slings, and other devices.

Help transfer patients to wheelchairs.

8:00 A.M.–9:00 A.M.

Direct or help patients to breakfast area. Set up feeding devices.

Help with serving and preparing patients' food trays. Help with feeding as necessary.

Remove and return food trays. Clean and put away personal eating devices.

Finish with morning care and baths and help with toilet needs.

9:00 A.M.–10:00 A.M.

Take a 15-minute coffee break at assigned time. Report to the charge nurse and your relief co-worker before leaving. Relieve your co-worker when he or she has coffee break.

Distribute clean linen to all your patients.

Working on one unit at a time:

Strip and remake beds.

Clean units.

Replace equipment.

Put away and check patients' clothing.

Give out fresh water.

Help patients to and from appointments.

10:00 A.M. – 1:00 P.M.
Collect and test urine specimens of diabetic patients.
Help patients with toilet needs and preparations for eating.
Go to lunch at assigned time. Report to charge nurse and your relief co-worker before going.
Replace your relief co-worker when she goes to lunch.
Direct or help able patients to dining area.
Help feed patients.

1:00 P.M.–3:00 P.M.
Prepare patients for rest period.
Answer signal lights.
Do special assignments such as cleaning storage closets.
Check and tidy your patients' rooms and bathrooms.
Help patients up from rest and straighten beds.

3:00 P.M.–3:30 P.M.
Report on your patients to the charge nurse.
Report on the completion of or problems with special assignments.
Report off duty to the charge nurse.
Sign out.

THE DOCTOR AND YOU

When you work in a nursing home or nursing service, you may be asked to help a doctor with physical examinations, diagnostic tests, and treatments. If a doctor asks you to help him and you do not understand what he is about to do, tell him that you will get someone else to help. If you have the time, however, watch the doctor and the person who assists him while they carry out the procedure. Ask them to teach you while they are working. Most doctors and members of a nursing staff are very helpful in this respect. In addition, many nursing homes and nursing services have in-service programs designed to teach staff members the procedures of that particular nursing facility so that the general education of all personnel is advanced.

When you care for a geriatric patient at home, a doctor will expect you to carry out all his orders for treatments and medications, to keep an accurate record of the patient's condition, and to tell him of any changes in condition that might need his attention.

You should protect the patient and yourself by requesting the doctor to write out and sign any order for special treatment or for a medication that does not require a prescription. If the doctor gives an order over the telephone, write it out exactly as he tells it to you. Then have him sign the order when he visits the patient.

See "Patient's Chart" in Chapter 2 and "To Give Medicines at Home" in Chapter 15.

If one of your duties is to take the patient to his doctor's office or to a clinic, be sure you take with you any information, specimens, and identification, such as the patient's Medicare and clinic cards, that might be needed.

THE SPECIALIST

All physicians are medical doctors, or M.D.'s, but some specialize in a single area of patient care. Doctors who specialize in the care of geriatric patients are called gerontologists or geriatricians.

Here is a list of other specialty titles and services that a geriatric patient might require.

Title of Doctor	Service		Doctor's Function
Allergist	Allergy		treats abnormal reactions to foods, pollens, dusts, and other substances
Anesthesiologist	Anesthesiology	(Anesth)	gives anesthesia
Cardiologist	Cardiology	(Card)	treats the heart and blood vessels
Dermatologist	Dermatology	(Derm)	treats skin
General Practitioner	General Practice	(GP)	treats all kinds of illnesses
Gynecologist	Gynecology	(GYN)	treats the female organs
Internist	Internal Medicine	(Med)	treats adults with medical problems
Neurosurgeon, Neurologist	Neurology	(Neuro)	treats the brain, spinal cord, and nervous system
Ophthalmologist	Ophthalmology	(Eye)	treats the eye
Orthopedist	Orthopedics	(Ortho)	treats muscles and bones
Otolaryngologist	Otolaryngology	(ENT)	treats the ears, nose, and throat
Pathologist	Pathology	(Path)	examines body tissues to aid in diagnosis or treatment
Physiatrist	Rehabilitation		restores all possible body mobility after loss
Psychiatrist	Psychiatry	(Psych)	treats mental disorders
Radiologist	Radiology	(X-ray)	works with radioactive tests and treatments
Surgeon	Surgical	(Surg)	performs operations
Urologist	Urology	(GU)	treats the male reproductive organs and the urinary organs of both sexes

TELEPHONING THE DOCTOR

In the section "Speaking on the Telephone," you will find correct telephone techniques for general medical use. When you telephone a doctor or expect to receive a call from him about a patient who is under the doctor's care, however, you use special additional methods.

Before you telephone, have a pencil and pad ready to write down any instructions.

Have information about the patient up to date and ready for reference in the event the doctor asks questions about the patient's condition.

Write down and have at hand the following information:

1. Exactly which changes prompt you to call the doctor.
2. The time when the changes took place and how these changes differ from the patient's earlier condition.
3. What steps you took to relieve the patient.

Example:
> The changes and time:
> > At 9:15 A.M. the patient began to breathe very fast.
> > His pulse was fast and weak.

His face was gray and sweaty.

Temperature — R99⁶ Pulse — 120 Respirations — 34

The earlier condition and time:

At 8:00 A.M. Temperature Oral 98⁴ Pulse — 84 Respirations — 24

Patient appeared normal in every way.

He was cheerful and ate all his breakfast.

He had a large, soft bowel movement of dark brown feces (stool) after breakfast.

What you did for the patient's relief:

I raised the patient's head level.

I started oxygen by nasal cannula as ordered (p.r.n.). (*See* "Abbreviations and Terms Used in Geriatric Care" later in this chapter.)

After you call the doctor and reach him, his office, or his answering service, give the following information at once:

My name is - - - -. I am the Aide on duty with Mr. - - - - -, 563 West 96 Street, Apt. 4F, Tel. 633-0643. I am calling because of the following changes in Mr. - - - - -'s condition.

Then give all the facts that you have written down about the changes, the earlier condition, and anything you did to relieve the patient.

Listen carefully and write down any instructions given to you by the doctor, his office nurse, or the answering service. Ask questions if there is anything you do not understand.

Then carry out the instructions.

THE GERIATRIC PATIENT AND YOU

There are three things that you must consider when you care for any patient: his body, his mind, and his emotions. These things are so woven one into the other that they are inseparable. Change in one causes change of the others. All must have attention. But the body, mind, and emotions of each person differ, and these differences are dependent on many factors, including the following:

Sex and age

The general health of the patient

His history of past illness

His nationality, race, religion, and income

His disposition, habits, and personality

His social background of relatives and friends

Whether he has ever been hospitalized

UNDERSTANDING AGING

Aging begins as soon as a baby is born. Even then, cells wear out and the body replaces them with new cells. In childhood and youth, the body's ability to make new cells is greater than the breakdown of old cells and so body growth occurs.

As life goes on, the ability to build cells and the breakdown of cells reach a balance. Body growth stops but the body is maintained.

This balance lasts only a short while before breakdown of cells exceeds the body's ability to replace them. More and more signs of aging occur as the ability to make new cells decreases.

Aging then is a normal process that causes progressive impairments in the functioning of the body, mind, and emotional makeup of any person. These impairments force the older person to give up more and more of his independence. They may threaten his place of respect within his family, business, and social affairs.

As part of the aging process, a geriatric patient usually develops a number of chronic, or continuing, diseases, such as diabetes or arthritis. He must learn to accept these conditions and to live with them in the most satisfactory way. To do this, he may need treatments, and he may have to use special equipment. He may also have to learn new ways to take care of himself, may have to endure pain, and may be restricted from former pleasures. Any of these things can be discouraging. The geriatric patient, therefore, needs constant encouragement to meet the challenges of aging.

He seldom has the drive of youth to help him. The ambitions and competitive feelings of younger years often are replaced by a withdrawal into himself. He may have a need for security and even for dependence. Recovery from a mild illness can be slowed by reluctance to return to the struggles of life. Yet his desire to live is a strong force that you can use to encourage him.

You should be aware of the medical goals of geriatric care. They are:

    To maintain the structure of individual life
    To promote the ability to handle stress
    To help the patient reach and keep maximal physical and mental abilities

You should also be aware of the emotional stress brought about by the conditions of aging. These are psychic blows and fears that affect the patient's health. They are:

    Becoming dependent
    Losing the respect of society
    Losing self-respect
    Losing the use of his senses, his abilities, and his mind
    Being abandoned by loved ones
    Adjusting to a new environment that requires him to give up some of his personal freedoms, belongings, position in his family and society, and habits, routines, and customs
    Dying

It is important for you to realize that a major adjustment is required for an elderly person to enter a nursing home. An adjustment is necessary regardless of whether the geriatric patient enters the home of his own choice or the choice of his family or a social agency.

You must understand that he may express his fears by withdrawing, being irritable or hostile, losing his appetite, or losing control of his bladder or bowel function.

You must do all that you can to lessen his fears, to make him feel secure and wanted, and to make him feel "at home" in a nursing home.

You can do this by:

    Encouraging and helping him to be as independent as possible
    By showing him respect and courtesy in every way
    By encouraging him to efforts that will make him proud of himself
    By teaching and encouraging him in the use of adaptive aids, such as crutches and hearing aids, that compensate for some of his losses
    By showing him that you genuinely care about him
    By helping him to adjust to the changes in his environment and respecting his freedoms, belongings, habits, routines, and customs

THE GERIATRIC PATIENT'S FAMILY AND YOU

You can also help the nursing home resident by understanding the sometimes trying behavior of family members. They often feel guilty about putting the patient in a home. They might feel grief that the patient requires more care than they can provide at home. Some feel inadequate.

It is not unusual for such family members to act in ways that can distress patient and staff. They may visit the patient too often or not at all. They may make unreasonable and unnecessary demands on the nursing staff, such as insisting that someone be at the patient's side 24 hours of every day. They may make unrealistic demands on the patient, such as insisting that he must walk after recovery from a stroke.

Understanding their thoughts and feelings can help you to relate to family members. Your patience and reassurance can soothe them and help remove their pressures from the patient and staff.

Family behavior is discussed at nursing staff meetings and at evaluations. Methods of coping with individual family behavior problems are designed and put into effect. As the patient adjusts to the nursing home, as he becomes interested, involved and "at home," family problems are usually resolved.

A GERIATRIC WHO'S WHO

Geriatric patient care is the result of teamwork. As a geriatric aide you work with many people, each of whom has one or more special duties and has taken special training either at school or on the job to prepare for his role on the team.

Activities of Daily Living (A.D.L.) Therapist has specialized knowledge and experience in retraining patients to take care of their body needs.

Dentist has specialized knowledge and experience in care of the teeth.

Dietitian plans the meals for hospitalized patients. This person has studied in an approved school for several years.

Doctor (M.D.) orders all routine and specific care for a patient. He is legally responsible for every medication and treatment that he orders. He goes through four years of college, four years of medical school, two years of internship at a hospital, and passes state examinations before he can practice.

Head or **Charge Nurse** is a registered nurse (R.N.) who is responsible for the safety and full care of all patients in an area. The charge nurse makes out the daily assignments for all R.N.'s, licensed practical nurses (L.P.N.'s), and aides who work in that area. She has advanced to this position through experience and on-the-job training.

Inhalation Therapist has specialized knowledge and experience in using certain gases to relieve patients with respiratory diseases.

Licensed Practical Nurse (L.P.N.) has studied one to two years in an approved nursing course and has passed state examinations on all subjects studied. (State examinations for L.P.N.'s are different from those for R.N.'s.)

Occupational Therapist plans and assists in the diversion and job training that help a patient to adjust to his illness. This therapist has completed an approved course of special training.

Pharmacist prepares and distributes to the charge nurses all medications used within a hospital. The pharmacist has a college degree and has studied at least two years in an approved school of pharmacy.

Physical Therapist directs and assists in the exercise of patients with poor nerve and muscle function. This person has passed an approved training program.

Podiatrist has specialized knowledge and experience in care of the feet.

Recreational Therapist provides entertainment and social functions for patients.

Registered Nurse (R.N.) has studied four years in a college nursing program and three full years at a hospital school or two years in an associate degree program at a community college. A registered nurse has passed state examinations on all subjects studied.

Social Worker helps the patient and his family to resolve problems resulting from the illness.

Speech Therapist   has specialized knowledge and experience in retraining patients with speech difficulties.

Superintendent or **Director of Nursing Services**   is responsible for all the nursing care given in the hospital, for the adequate staffing of the hospital, and for the conduct, hiring, and firing of all employees who give nursing care. The superintendent usually has several university degrees as well as a nursing diploma from a hospital.

Technician   does special work, such as laboratory analysis of specimens, and operates equipment, such as an x-ray machine. This person has passed a special training course and often has had on-the-job training.

Volunteers   are people who offer free services to help others.

A GERIATRIC WHO IS WHERE

A geriatric nursing facility offers many services for older people. Every facility, whether nursing home or day care center, may not have the space or money to provide special rooms and equipment for all the services in the following list. A facility can arrange to provide the services, however, either by taking patients outside the facility to governmental, community, or private services or by bringing practitioners of services into the nursing facility. Here are some areas of service that you should know and locate.

Activities Office   an office for planning and arranging recreational and social activities.

A.D.L. Room   a place where training in activities of daily living is given to patients.

Auditorium   a large room used for entertainment, large social gatherings, and any activity requiring space.

Barber Shop   provides grooming services to male residents.

Beauty Parlor   provides grooming services to female residents.

Central Supply   supplies all areas of a nursing home with equipment and provisions.

Chapel   a place for private prayer and religious services.

Coffee Shop   serves beverages and snacks to residents and guests.

Dentist's Office   an area equipped to give dental care to residents.

Diet Kitchen   a separate kitchen area where meals are prepared for patients on special diets.

Doctor's Office   usually the office of the head doctor or of the resident doctor at the nursing home.

Eye, Ear, Nose, and Throat Clinic   an area equipped to give examinations and treatments to these parts of the body.

Housekeeping   the office and equipment center for personnel responsible for the overall cleanliness of the nursing home.

Inhalation Room   a place where gases and machines used in giving inhalation therapy are stored.

In-service Education   an office and classroom where instruction is given to personnel.

Intensive Care Unit   an area equipped and staffed to give concentrated nursing care and emergency services.

Laboratories   areas equipped to test and examine body fluids and tissues.

Library   an area equipped with books and other reading material.

Maintenance   the office and storage area for those who maintain and repair the building and its furnishings.

Medical Clinic   an area equipped for medical examination and treatments.

Morgue   a storage area for the body of a person who has died.

Nurses Station   a desk area equipped with patient care records and a call system through which each patient can communicate with nursing personnel. A medicine closet is also a part of the station.

Occupational Therapy (O.T.)   a specially equipped area where patients can learn and practice an occupation for therapeutic purposes.

Pharmacy an area equipped to supply the medicine needed by patients.
Physical Therapy (P.T.) an area equipped for treatment by stimulation of body activity.

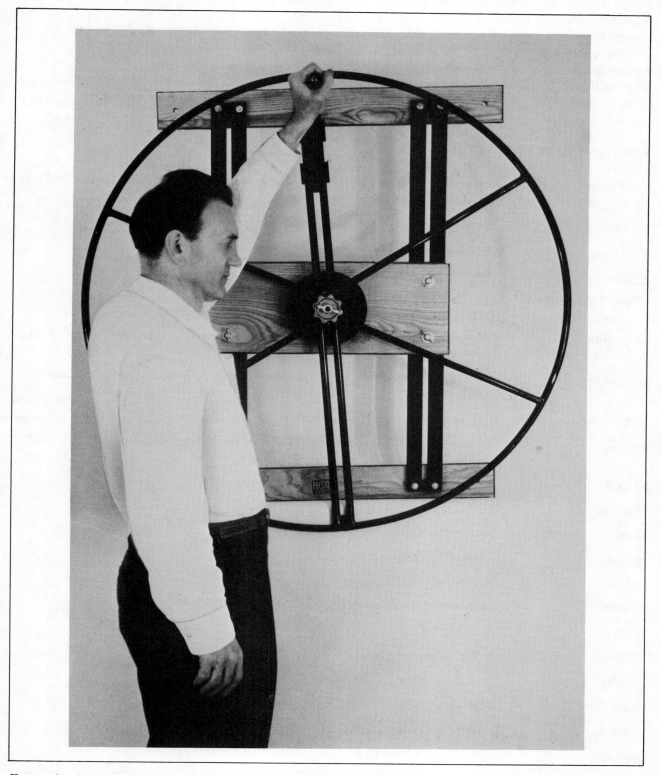

Figure 1. A wheel for arm exercising in a physical therapy (P.T.) room. (Reprinted by permission of J. A. Preston Corp.,© 1971.)

Podiatry   an area equipped for a specialist in foot care to treat patients.
Recreation Room   an area equipped for patients to play games.
Social Service   an office for social workers.
Solarium   An area glass-enclosed to allow the sun to enter.
Special Care Unit   an area equipped and staffed to give care to patients who are unable to care for themselves.
Sundry Store   an area where patients can shop for small personal items and gifts.
Visiting Room   An area equipped with chairs where patients can visit with guests and each other.
X-ray or **Radiation**   an area equipped to take x-ray pictures and give radiation treatment.

WORDS USED IN GERIATRIC CARE

abduction	movement of a part of the body away from an imaginary midline. (*See* "Range of Motion Exercise.")
abrasion	a rubbing away or scraping of the skin.
abscess	a localized collection of pus in a cavity.
acute	sudden and severe.
adaptive equipment	things such as a hearing aid or long-handled tongs that allow a patient to regain use of a body part or to perform a body function.
adduction	movement of a part of the body toward an imaginary midline. (*See* "Range of Motion Exercise.")
allergic reaction	an abnormal reaction to a substance, such as pollens, certain foods, and medications.
ambulatory	not bedridden. Able to walk.
anemia	reduction in the number of red cells, of the hemoglobin content, or of both, in the blood.
anterior	front.
antidote	a remedy for poisoning.
anus	the outlet for the rectum.
aphasia	loss of the ability to speak.
arthritis	a painful inflammation of joints.
atrophy	wasting or lessening of ability.
axilla	armpit.
bacteria	microscopic organisms.
bladder	a hollow organ in which urine collects.
bland diet	soft food, without spice and roughage.
buttocks	fleshy areas of the lower part of the back that cover the hip joints.
cardiac	pertaining to the heart.
cataract	condition of the eye that impairs vision.

ON BEING A GERIATRIC AIDE

catheterize	to introduce a sterile tube into the bladder to withdraw urine.
Cheyne-Stokes	a type of respiration that often precedes death.
chronic	of long duration.
circulatory system	movement of the blood through the heart, veins, arteries, and capillaries.
colostomy	an operation by which the large intestine is made to open onto the abdomen.
coma	a state of unconsciousness.
compound fracture	a broken bone protruding through the skin.
condom	a rubber sheath worn on the penis in urinary drainage.
contaminated	in the presence of germs.
contusion	a bruise.
convulsion	involuntary spasms or contractions of big muscles.
cyanosis	a blueness of the skin due to a lack of oxygen.
cystitis	an inflammation of the urinary bladder.
cystoscope	an instrument used to examine the interior of the urinary system.
debilitated	extremely weakened.
decubitus ulcer	a pressure sore or ulcer.
defecation	the discharge of feces. Also called *bowel movement*.
dehydration	a condition resulting from severe loss of fluids from the body.
depression	a state of morbid unhappiness.
dermatitis	an inflammation of the skin.
diabetes	a disease caused by the inability of the body to produce enough insulin, a glandular secretion.
diagnosis	determination of the patient's condition or the cause of an illness.
diarrhea	frequent loose or watery stools.
digital stimulation	finger massage of the anus to induce a bowel movement.
dislocation	the displacement of a bone.
disoriented	in a confused state of mind.
edema	the accumulation of fluid in the tissues.
elimination	the process of getting rid of body wastes.
emaciation	a wasted, lean body condition.
emesis	vomiting.
epilepsy	a nervous disease marked by recurring convulsions and loss of consciousness.
evaluation	determination of physical, mental, and emotional health.
excrete	discharge waste matter.
extension	straightening a part of the body.

THE QUALITIES OF A GERIATRIC AIDE

feces	the excretion of the bowels. Also called *stool*.
femur	a bone extending from the hip to the knee.
flatus	intestinal gas.
flexion	bending a part of the body.
gastric	pertaining to the stomach.
genitalia	the external sex organs of the male or female.
geriatrics	the study and care of elderly persons.
gynecology	the study of female reproduction, sex organs, and their diseases.
hematoma	a darkened area of the skin containing blood.
hemiplegia	paralysis of one side of the body.
hemorrhage	the escape of blood from a blood vessel.
hemorrhoids	piles. Varicose veins of the anus or rectum.
hernia	a weakness in a muscle wall that allows an inner body part to break through it.
hydrotherapy	treatment by water (Fig. 2).

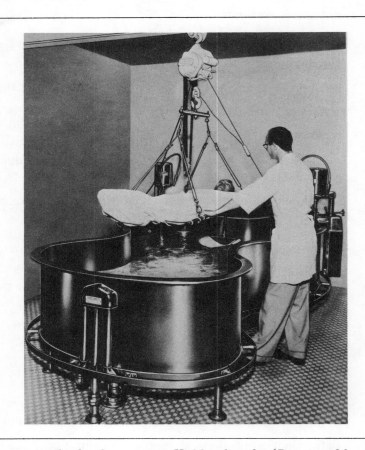

Figure 2.   A patient receiving hydrotherapy in a Hubbard tank. (Reprinted by permission of © J. A. Preston Corp., 1971.)

ON BEING A GERIATRIC AIDE

hypertension	high blood pressure.
immunization	the process of making a person less susceptible to a disease.
incontinence	inability to control the elimination of feces or urine.
infection	the invasion of body tissues by disease organisms.
inflammation	a condition characterized by redness, pain, heat, and swelling.
inhalation	the drawing of air or other vapors into the lungs.
isolation	the separation of one person (or object) from others.
Medicaid	a program in which federal, state, and sometimes local governments share the costs of certain medical services.
Medicare	a federal program in which certain health insurance benefits are given to people who are 65 or older.
mental health	the state of being able to function under ordinary daily pressures without feeling great fears, confusion, or nervousness.
obesity	fatness.
orthesis	braces or other devices placed on the body for the treatment of a physical disability.
pallor	paleness.
paralysis	loss of the ability to move, or to feel sensation in, a body part.
passive exercise	the movement of a person's body by a force outside of himself (by another person or a machine).
penis	the male sex organ.
physiotherapy	diagnosis and treatment with heat, massage, and manipulation.
posterior	back.
prone	lying face down.
prostatectomy	removal of the prostate gland in the male.
prosthesis	an artificial replacement for a missing part of the body.
rectum	the last 8–10 inches of the large intestine.
rehabilitation	methods used to return use of body parts after loss.
remotivation	renewal of interest in living.
resident	a patient who lives in a nursing home or other institution.
resocialization	renewal of interest in being with other people.
restraint	a binder to prevent self-injury. (Fig. 3).
scrotum	the genital sac of the male.
sedative	a medication that calms an excited patient.
self-care	the ability to dress, groom, and feed oneself.

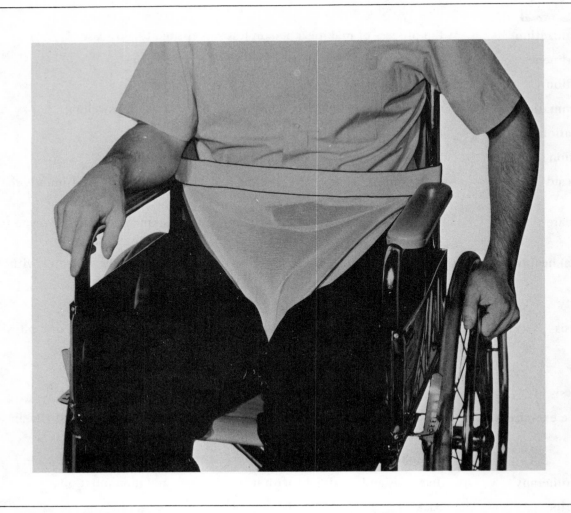

Figure 3. A wheelchair restraint. (By permission of © J. T. Posey Co.)

senile	pertaining to old age.
shock	an upset caused by inadequate blood circulation resulting in lowered blood pressure, a rapid, weak pulse, and pale, clammy skin.
stool	feces. A bowel movement.
supine	lying face up.
testicles (testes)	two male reproductive glands located in the scrotum.
therapeutic	relating to the treatment of disease.
transfer	move from one location to another (*Example*: from bed to wheelchair).
umbilicus	the navel or belly button.
ureter	one of two tubes leading from the kidneys to the urinary bladder.
urethra	the tube leading from the urinary bladder to the surface of the body.

ON BEING A GERIATRIC AIDE

uterus	the female organ in which the embryo develops.
Velcro fastener	a self-sticking type of clothes fastener.
voiding	urinating.
vulva	the external female sex organs.

ABBREVIATIONS AND TERMS USED IN GERIATRIC CARE

Doctors, nurses, and other medical personnel use special terms and abbreviations that are not common outside the medical field. You will need to learn what they mean. Those explained here are the ones you will use most often in your work as a geriatric aide.

a.c.	before meals	NPO	nothing by mouth
Amb	ambulatory	NS	normal saline
anti-	against (as antidote)	o.d.	once a day
b.i.d.	twice a day	OOB	out of bed
b.i.w.	twice a week	OPD	outpatient department
BM	bowel movement	oz.	ounce
BP	blood pressure	p.c.	after meals
BR	bed rest	pMn	after midnight
BRP	bathroom privileges	PO	by mouth
c̄ or c	with	post-	after (as "postoperative")
caps	capsule	pre-	before (as "preoperative")
CCU	coronary care unit	p.r.n.	as required, whenever necessary
contra-	against (as "contraindicated")	q.d.	every day
CBR	complete bed rest	q.4h.	every four hours
CVA	cerebrovascular accident or stroke	q.i.d.	four times a day
D.K.	diet kitchen	q.m.	every morning
D/W	dextrose in water	q.n.	every night
ENT	ears, nose, and throat	q.o.d.	every other day
ER	emergency room	q.w.	every week
GI	gastrointestinal	ROM	range of motion
GP	general practitioner	s̄	without
gt, gtt	drop, drops	SSE	soapsuds enema
GU	genitourinary	stat.	at once, immediately
GYN	gynecology	t.	teaspoon
h.s.	at bedtime	T.	tablespoon
I & O	intake and output	tab	tablet
ICU	intensive care unit	t.i.d.	three times a day
IV	intravenous	TPR	temperature, pulse, respiration
MOM	milk of magnesia	URI	upper respiratory infection
n & d	night and day	wt & ht	weight and height

noc   night

q̄ every

MEASUREMENTS USED IN GERIATRIC CARE

The following table for liquids is approximate. One liter is not the exact equivalent of one quart, but is 1.056 quarts, and a pint of all liquids does not weigh exactly a pound. It is sufficiently accurate, however, for all but the most precise measurements.

cc.	cubic centimeter	ml.	milliliter
ft. or '	foot	oz.	ounce
in. or "	inch	pt.	pint
L.	liter	qt.	quart
lb.	pound	yd.	yard

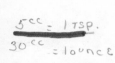

5 cc = 1 TSP.
30 cc = 1 ounce

1 ml. = 1 cc.
30 ml. = 30 cc. = 1 oz.
250 ml. = 240 cc. = 8 oz. = 1 measuring cup
500 ml. = 480 cc. = 16 oz. = 1 pt.
1000 ml. = 950 cc. = 32 oz. = 1 qt.
(or 1 L.)

3 t. = 1 T.
1 pt. = 1 lb.

12 in. = 1 ft.
18" = 1-1/2'
36 in. = 3 ft. = 1 yd.

Part II

Meeting Your Geriatric Patient's Needs

2

THE COMMON NEEDS OF GERIATRIC PATIENTS

STUDY GUIDE

What are the needs of all geriatric patients?

What needs do geriatric patients share with all other humans?

What is routine care?

What is specific care?

Who orders both the routine and the specific care for a patient?

What four things are part of an overall care plan for a geriatric patient?

What is an evaluation? A reevaluation?

How often is a reevaluation done?

What tests are done before evaluation or reevaluation?

Who takes part in an evaluation or reevaluation?

What are the three parts of the nursing care plan for a geriatric patient?

Why is self-care important?

Why are activities important?

What is the first duty in geriatric nursing care?

What are the four levels of geriatric nursing care?

Tell six things the doctor may order in routine care for a patient.

What may be included in the doctor's orders for specific care of a patient?

What is a nameplate?

What is a patient's chart?

What sheets are in a patient's chart?

What is a cardex?

What is an assignment sheet?

What are intake and output sheets?

Tell how to keep a record on a patient at home.

THE NEEDS OF ALL GERIATRIC PATIENTS

Although their health conditions vary from vigor to complete dependence, all geriatric patients have certain common needs. These are:

    To live and enjoy life as long as possible
    To be relieved of hard work and protected from health hazards
    To have skills, rights, and social standing protected and encouraged and to have property
        protected
    To remain active in affairs of life and society
    To die in dignity and comfort

Routine Care

Physical
Sicological
Social
Religious
Finical
Sovual

There are other needs that geriatric patients share with all humans. They are:
    Body warmth
    Air to breath
    Exercise
    Body cleanliness
    Food
    To get rid of body wastes
    Sleep
In nursing, meeting these needs is called *routine care*.

Specific Care

Besides those needs shared with others, a patient has individual needs that develop because of his health.

Example: A person with diabetes might need the following:
Laboratory tests to determine the sugar content of his blood and urine.
Medicine to control the sugar level in the blood and urine.
A special diet to control the intake of foods that affect the sugar level in the blood and urine.

In nursing, meeting these needs is called *specific care*.

THE DOCTOR ORDERS A PATIENT'S CARE

The doctor always orders both the routine and the specific care for a patient. Since aging causes progressive changes in a person, the doctor expects a geriatric patient to require increasing amounts of specific care. The doctor, therefore, orders an overall care plan for the patient. This care plan is designed to help personnel do the following:

    Recognize early signs of change.
    Prepare to meet needs of change.
    Support the patient during changes.
    Help the patient adjust to changes once they occur.

The doctor makes a care plan after examining the patient and meeting with others who are involved in the care of the patient. He changes the care plan when the needs of the patient change.

EVALUATION AND REEVALUATION

An *evaluation* is a first determination of a patient's needs based on up-to-date information about him. This information includes health, family, social, religious, and economic histories.

A *reevaluation* is any later determination of a patient's needs based on a review of previous information about him and new information.

In a nursing facility, a patient is evaluated shortly after admission. Regular reevaluation may be scheduled once or twice a year, or more often if a patient's condition seems to require it. An unscheduled reevaluation may be called at the request of staff members if a patient's needs change in marked, unexpected ways.

Tests done before evaluation or reevaluation help to determine the patient's immediate condition. The patient's previous condition, the orders of his doctor, the time lapse since his last evaluation, and the policy of the nursing home affect the choice of tests. They may be some or all of the following:

Laboratory tests
urine
blood
others (such as sputum) as indicated by a specific condition

General physical examination
Special eye tests
vision
glaucoma (a serious condition caused by increased pressure of fluid within the eyeball)

Hearing
Foot
Dental
Muscle function
Activities of daily living (A.D.L.)
Psychiatric
X-rays
chest
others (such as hip, after fracture) as indicated by a specific condition

Speech

During the Evaluation

Depending on the policy of the nursing home or facility, and on the condition of the patient, some or all of the following staff members might attend an evaluation or reevaluation:

Geriatrician or patient's own doctor
Physiatrist
Psychiatrist
Nursing supervisor
Day nurses and aides who have direct care of patient
Social worker
Physical therapist
A.D.L. therapist
Occupational therapist

During the evaluation or reevaluation, reports of the preevaluation tests are considered along with reports on the patient by those present. If possible, the patient attends and is questioned about his complaints and problems. Then, the doctor orders any necessary changes to be made in the patient's care plan.

THE PATIENT'S CARE PLAN

The care plan of a geriatric patient has three separate but interrelated parts:
Self-care
Activities
Nursing care

Self-Care

Some people think that showing concern for an elderly person means relieving him of all responsibilities and efforts. They argue that an old person has earned the right to do nothing and to have others wait on him. These people mean well, but they are wrong to confuse care with unnecessary service.

A geriatric patient should not exhaust himself, and he should have as much help as he needs. The word to remember is *needs*. He needs only that amount of help without which he could not function. Unnecessary assistance can harm him.

In self-care, the patient is provided with needed physical activity and with important feelings of independence and pride. Self-care helps him to remain alert to his surroundings and to prolong his life.

To encourage and maintain the patient's ability to perform self-care, his doctor orders a regular program of physical therapy. If the patient is physically handicapped, the doctor orders special equipment, such as a brace, walker, or wheelchair, that will keep the patient active. The doctor also orders training in activities of daily living, through which the patient learns new ways to help himself function. The doctor may order adaptive equipment that enables the patient to feed, dress, groom, and help himself in the bathroom.

Activities

Besides self-care, a patient needs other activities. He should have work to do that carries over from one day to the next. He should have opportunities to learn, and he should have a social and recreational life.

Occupational therapy trains the patient for and provides work. Depending on a patient's ability and interests, his participation in occupational therapy may range from full-time employment at a regular job to a few minutes spent on a simple craft.

Although occupational therapy may offer some learning experiences, a patient should have other chances to learn. Many nursing facilities offer classes, lectures, and field trips. They may encourage informal talks in which well-informed patients can share their knowledge with other patients.

Sometimes learning is combined with social and recreational activities. Theater programs and concerts may be made available. Games, parties, and events are planned.

The intent of all activities is to involve the patient as much as possible, to keep him interested, to keep him active, and to keep him in the mainstream of life.

Nursing Care

Nursing is the last part of a geriatric care plan to be mentioned here. This does not mean that nursing is less important than self-care or activities. It does mean that the first duty in geriatric nursing is to cooperate with and enforce self-care and activity programs.

Four Levels of Nursing Care

Because of the wide range in the specific needs of geriatric patients, care in a nursing home is divided into four levels. Most nursing homes have a separate area for each kind of care, equipped and staffed according to the needs of the patient at that level of care. These levels are:

1. *Independent resident.* This patient lives at a nursing home in much the same way as a person might live at a hotel. He requires a minimum of nursing care and is able to take complete care of himself.

2. *Resident who requires continual medical supervision.* This patient may have one or more conditions that require regular observation, treatment, and medication. He might, for example, have a heart condition or severe arthritis.

3. *Resident who is temporarily acutely ill.* This patient may be a resident from any of the other three areas who has developed an illness, such as flu, and who requires concentrated nursing care for a short time.

4. *Resident who is chronically disoriented.* This patient suffers from brain damage and requires total care.

How Nursing Care is Ordered

For Routine Care

The doctor writes orders that tell the following information about the patient's routine care.

1. The doctor orders which vital signs to observe and when to do it. (Vital signs are temperature, pulse, respirations, and blood pressure.) He might order:

> TPR q.d. – Temperature, pulse, and respirations once every day
> TPR q.4h. – Temperature, pulse, and respirations every four hours, day and night
> BP q.w. – Blood pressure once every week
> BP q.2h. – Blood pressure every two hours, day and night

2. The doctor orders the patient's activity. He would order one of the following:

> CBR – Complete bed rest
> BR – Bed rest
> OOB – Out of bed
> Amb – Ambulatory or walking
> BRP – Bathroom privileges
> Up in chair

3. The doctor orders the kind of bath the patient can have. Sometimes this is understood in the order for activity.

> CBR implies a bed bath and occupied bed
> BR implies a partial bath and occupied bed
> OOB and Amb imply a tub bath or shower and open bed
> BRP – Needs special order for bath or shower but open bed.
> Up in chair – Needs special order for bath or shower but open bed.

4. The doctor orders the patient's diet or food. He would order one of the following diets:
   Regular
   Soft
   Clear liquid
   Full liquid
   Special diet or Diet Kitchen (D.K.)

5. The doctor orders what the patient may require for good bowel and urine function. He might order the following:
   A laxative — MOM oz. ii q.n., h.s. (milk of magnesia, ounces 2, every night, at bedtime)
   An enema — SSE, q.o.d., p.r.n. (soapsuds enema, every other day, when necessary)
   Increased fluid intake — Force fluids
   Measure fluids taken in and urine voided — I & O (intake and output)

6. The doctor orders a sleeping medication if necessary. He might order:
   Phenobarbital ½, h.s., p.r.n. (phenobarbital ½, at bedtime, as needed)

For Specific Care

Besides the routine care, the doctor orders any examinations, tests, treatments, medications, equipment, and therapy that he may want the particular patient to have. He might order one or more of the following as well as many other things:
   Defer (or hold) in A.M. — hold breakfast until after blood tests or other tests are done
   Walker — patient is to use a special walking aid
   Whirlpool, q.d., 20 min. L leg — patient's left leg is to be given treatment in a whirlpool machine for 20 minutes each day (Fig. 4)
   O_2 stat. — start oxygen at once
   Urine for glucose a.c., t.i.d. — test urine for sugar content before meals, three times a day
   S.T., q.d. — speech therapy every day

THE PROFESSIONAL NURSING STAFF SEES THAT ORDERS ARE CARRIED OUT

The professional nurses have the responsibility for carrying out the orders that a doctor writes for each patient. In order to simplify the carrying out of the orders, and to double check on all orders being carried out, the nurses transfer all orders to the following:
   Patient's chart
   Cardex (medicine and treatment cards)
   Request slips to different departments, such as x-ray and labs
   Diet slips to the kitchen
   Assignment sheet or assignment blackboard
   Intake and output sheets

Nameplate and Addressograph

The Addressograph is a machine used to stamp important information about the patient on every piece of chart paper or test sheet needed for the patient. The nameplate includes the patient's name, admission date, sex, religion, hospital or nursing home number, and doctor's name.

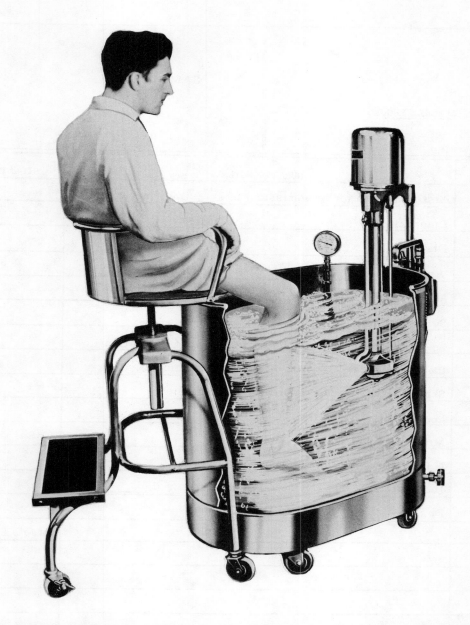

Figure 4. A patient using whirlpool treatment. (Reprinted by permission of © J. A. Preston Corp., 1971.)

Patient's Chart

A chart is kept on every patient in a nursing home. The chart is a permanent record of a patient's progress. The makeup of a chart differs from one nursing home to another, but it usually contains:

- Admission Sheet (Fig. 5)
- Physician's Order Sheet
- Physician's Notes (on patient's progress)
- Temperature, Pulse, and Respirations Sheet
- Nurses' Notes (on patient's progress. Fig. 6)
- Laboratory Test Results
- A.D.L. (or other special examination and treatment sheets)
- Evaluation and Reevaluation Sheets

SAMPLE

NURSES RECORD

DATE TIME	NURSES NOTES	SIGNATURE
10-1-70	First admission (or re-admission) of a _____ yr. old via _____	
	Diagnosis: Onset:	
	Disability: B.D.	
	Vital Signs: Hgt. _____ Wgt.	
	Allergies:	
	Seizures:	
	Bowel: (Incontinent – Regulated with type of medication)	
	Bladder: (Foley – Condom – Control – Incontinent)	
	Skin: (Clear – reddened areas – decubitus)	
	Appliances:	
	Medications:	
	A.D.L. (transfer – dressing – feeding)	
	Locker # _____ 50¢ deposit received _____	
	Dr. _____ notified	
		Nurse's Signature
	-4-	

Figure 5. Admission sheet.

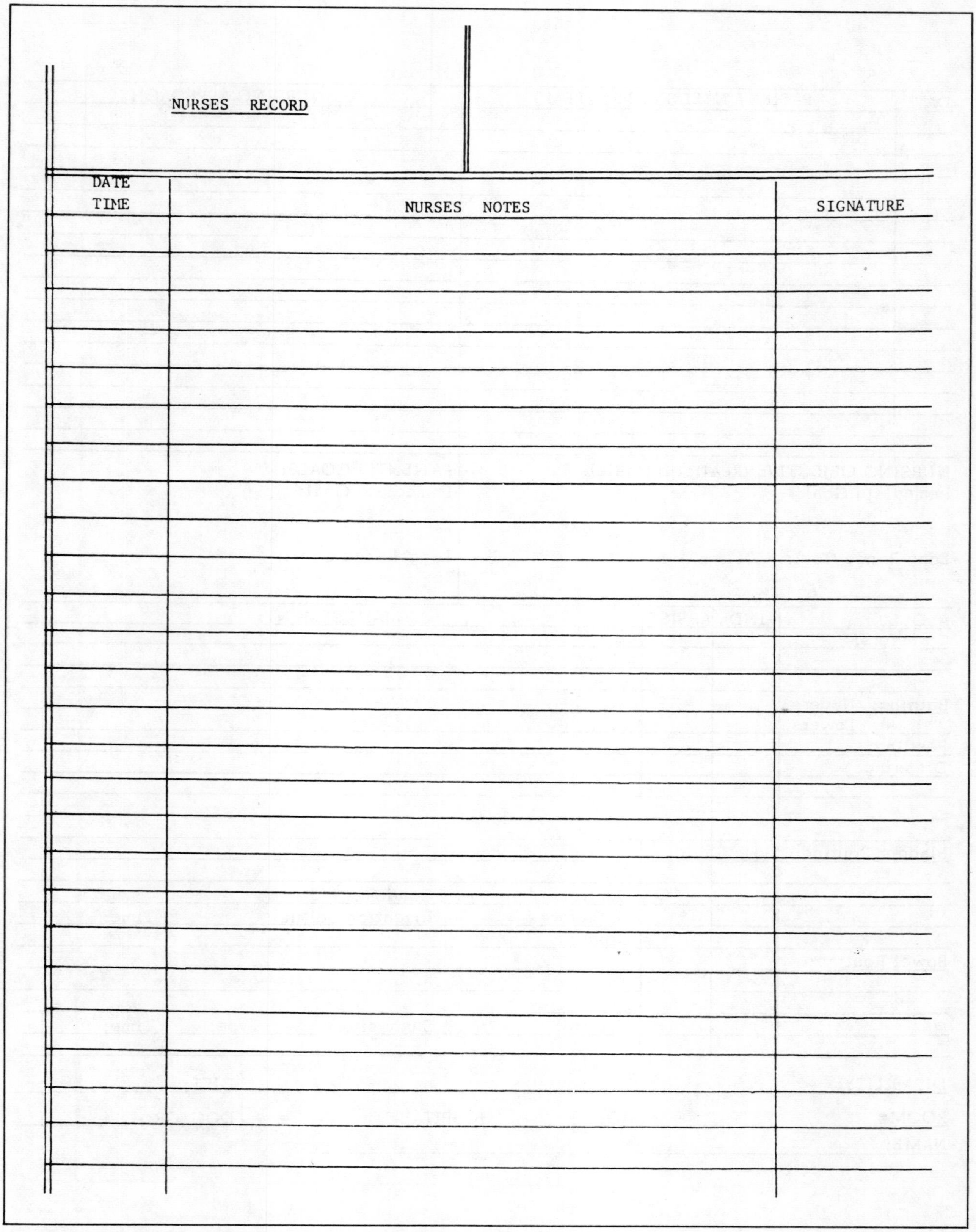

DATE TIME	NURSES NOTES	SIGNATURE

NURSES RECORD

Figure 6. Nurses' continuing note sheet.

DATE	PATIENT NEEDS or PROBLEMS	NURSING APPROACH

NURSING OBJECTIVE (Realistic Goals):
Immediate Goal:

Long Range Goal:

PATIENT'S GOALS:
Immediate Goal:

Long Range Goal:

A.D.L.	IND	ASSIST	MANAGEMENT:
Transfers:			
Bathing: Uppers			
Lowers			
Feeding:			
Dressing:			
Bladder Routine:			
			Control: Condom:
			Catheter# Irrigation Sol'n: Time:
			Crede:
Bowel Routine:			
			Control: Suppository: Type: Time:

DISABLEITY: _____   DIET: _____

ROOM# _____   AGE: _____   HOSPITAL# _____   DOCTOR: _____

NAME: _____

Figure 7. Cardex.

MEETING YOUR GERIATRIC PATIENT'S NEEDS

DATE	MEDICATION	TIME	D/C	DATE	TREATMENT	TIMES

THE COMMON NEEDS OF GERIATRIC PATIENTS

The patient's chart remains at the desk of the area of level of care to which the patient is assigned and it is transferred with him if he moves to another level of care.

Cardex

This is a portable, open filing case that holds a card for each patient assigned to an area. A patient's card contains all his medicine and treatment orders (Fig. 7). It is only necessary to check the cardex to see what routine or specific orders any patient must receive.

Assignment Sheet

This is a sheet that is made out by the charge nurse dividing all the work that must be done in one area among the workers present. Each R.N., L.P.N., aide, attendant, or orderly is given a number of patients to care for, as well as other duties. The care for each patient is listed under that patient's name and room number.

Example:
September 9, 1973
Aide — Mary Smith
Assignment:

1. Thomas Jones — Rm. 301
   Nasal catheter O_2 continuous
   Keep head of bed elevated
   D.K. — Feed
   Side rails up
   Bed bath
   Intake and output
   SSE
2. Mrs. Jacob Silverstein — Rm. 304
   OOB
   Shower
   Test urine for sugar at every voiding
   Routine urine spec.
3. Give out 10:00 A.M. nourishment
4. Take TPRs

In some nursing facilities, an assignment blackboard is used instead of an assignment sheet. An assignment board is prepared by the charge nurse in a way similar to the preparation of an assignment sheet.

Intake and Output Sheets

These sheets are made out for each patient on measured intake and output. Intake sheets are usually taped to the bedside stand. Output sheets are usually posted on the wall of the bathroom, utility, or hopper room.

WHEN CARE IS GIVEN AT HOME

If you are at home with a patient, you should make sure that you follow a similar plan.

Keep a record on your patient. A loose-leaf book is good for this. Mark certain pages *Doctor's Orders* and have the doctor write in and sign any medication or treatment orders he gives for the patient.

Mark certain pages *Nursing Notes* and keep a record of changes in your patient's condition and the date, time, and results of all treatments.

Mark certain pages *Temperature, Pulse, and Respirations.* Keep a record of the date, time, and data for these vital signs.

Mark certain sheets *Daily Duties* and make out your own assignments.

Mark certain sheets *Intake and Output* (if your patient needs these) and keep an accurate record of his fluid balance.

3

YOUR GERIATRIC PATIENT NEEDS A CLEAN, SAFE, COMFORTABLE PLACE

STUDY GUIDE

Cleanliness

How is the long-term resident in a nursing home encouraged to think about his room?

When is an inventory taken of a resident's belongings?

What belongings of a resident can be removed without consent?

Why is environmental cleanliness so necessary for the aged?

Name four ways in which environmental cleanliness is provided for a patient.

What housekeeping duties are you expected to do as a geriatric aide?

How is a patient's personal laundry done?

What makes up a unit?

What equipment do you need to clean an occupied unit?

Tell what you would do to clean an occupied unit.

Tell what you would do to clean a patient's bathroom.

What should you remember when arranging the occupied unit of a geriatric patient?

When does a unit get a special cleaning and disinfection?

Tell how to clean and disinfect a unit.

What is sterile technique and when is it used?

Tell some ways to sterilize materials.

Tell some of the general rules about sterile technique.

Tell how to put on sterile gloves.

Tell how to handle sterile forceps.

Safety

How can you prevent accidents?

Why are special safety precautions necessary for geriatric patients?

Tell some safety precautions regarding the bed of a geriatric patient.

Tell some safety precautions regarding the clothing of a geriatric patient.

Tell some safety precautions concerning the bath of a geriatric patient.

Tell some safety precautions about the food of a geriatric patient.

Tell some safety precautions to observe in a room used by a geriatric patient.

Tell some safety precautions to observe in hallways used by geriatric patients.

A patient or resident in a geriatric nursing home is there for long-term care that often lasts for many years. On entering the home, the resident is assigned to a room or part of a room that he can expect to occupy during most of his remaining life. He is encouraged to think of this place as his home and to bring to it certain personal belonging that make him feel at ease. These may include: Clothing for all seasons, books, pictures, photographs, a radio, hobby equipment, and even a favorite chair or chest of drawers.

To accommodate such belongings, the residential units of a long-term geriatric home have more equipment and storage space than do usual nursing care units. In addition to the basic unit furnishings of bed, bedside stand, bed light, bedside chair, and wastebasket, many a residential unit has a chest of drawers with a dressing mirror, a large clothes closet, and a comfortable, armed sitting chair.

Care of the unit includes care of the furnishings and the patient's belongings. Clothing and other possessions should be examined regularly for wear or soil and cleaned or replaced as needed.

Many old people save or treasure seemingly unnecessary things. An inventory of a resident's belongings should be taken on admission and thereafter at regular intervals set by the charge nurse. Nothing belonging to a patient should be removed or replaced without the specific consent of the patient and the charge nurse. Sometimes the signature of the patient or a member of his family is needed before an item can be removed or replaced.

Many old people are forgetful and tend to misplace things. Organizing belongings in a systematic way helps both the patient and you to keep track of his belongings.

A special effort should be made with each patient to organize his unit in the best possible way to meet his specific needs and tastes. The unit of a hemiplegia patient, for example, should be organized so that his affected side is next to a wall and the bedside stand is available to his unaffected side.

Environmental cleanliness is more necessary for the aged than for the average adult. Greater precautions must be taken to prevent infection in a person whose resistance to disease is constantly changing. Greater precautions must be taken to prevent the transfer of infection from an infected patient to another person.

Cleanliness for a patient's environment is provided by:
> General cleanliness of the building.
> Particular cleanliness of the patient's unit.
> Sterilization and disinfection of certain articles or areas after use by one patient to prevent transfer of germs to another person.
> The use of sterile techniques in some of the treatment and care of the patient's internal body.

HOUSEKEEPING DUTIES DONE BY AIDES

YOU DO THIS

Give out linens and put them away.

Send soiled linens to the laundry.

Keep soap, paper cup, and paper towel dispensers filled.

Keep the utility and supply rooms clean and orderly.

Keep storage closets clean, orderly, and labeled.

Clean up and put away equipment after treatments and examinations.

Clean treatment trays and other equipment. See that each is supplied with everything it needs.

Keep wastebaskets empty.

Notice, and clean up, any spilled fluid or broken glass anywhere.

Keep the patients' units clean.

Help the patient keep his clothing and personal equipment clean and neat.

Report to the charge nurse if furniture or equipment is in poor working condition, if any light is not working, or if any mattress, pillow, drape, slipcover, patient screen, or other item is torn, worn, or stained.

Keep bathrooms and toilet equipment clean.

Patients' Personal Laundry

Many geriatric facilities have automatic washers and dryers conveniently located so that able patients can do their own personal laundry and aides can easily do the laundry of other patients.

STANDARD EQUIPMENT IN THE PATIENT'S UNIT

The Bed

A hospital bed has movable parts, which can be operated to position a patient. Several types of hospital beds are in use today, and you should be familiar with them all.

Handcrank: This is a waist-high bed with two handcranks at the foot. The upper portion of the bed is raised or lowered by turning one crank and the knee area of the bed is raised or lowered by turning the other. Bed rails can be attached.

Electric: This type is most commonly used in geriatric facilities. The electric bed is operated by pushing the buttons on a hand control box. The operation is so easy that the patient can position himself when that is desirable. This bed offers more positioning possibilities. As well as elevating the back and knees, the entire bed can be raised or tilted headward or footward. Nursing facilities that use electric beds usually enforce a safety policy. A bed must be kept in low position at all times except when someone is with the patient. Side rails are a part of the bed and these are raised and lowered by an easy-to-operate hand control. Many nursing homes require that side rails be raised on all beds at night and on the beds of confused or weak bed patients at all times.

Sometimes to allow self-help a trapeze is attached to a bed in such a way that it hangs securely within the patient's upreached grasp. If the patient pulls on the trapeze, he can help move himself about the bed.

The Bedside Stand

The stand is usually positioned next to the head of the bed so that the stand top and drawer are within the patient's easy reach. Belongings such as toothbrush and toothpaste, comb and brush, and drinking straws may be kept in the drawer. A small tray with a water pitcher and drinking glass is set on top of the stand. A bar on one side of the stand holds towels and washcloth. A cabinet that opens to the front holds personal equipment such as washbasin, soap dish, bedpan, urinal, etc.

All bedstand equipment is sterilized before use by a new patient, and it is cleaned and sterilized at regular intervals. Water pitchers and glasses are sterilized every day. Many nursing facilities use disposable pitchers and glasses. These are usually changed daily and have the added advantages of being light-weight and unbreakable.

The Lamp

An adjustable lamp is usually attached to the wall of the unit in a location that will give a good light for reading as well as for treatments and examinations.

The Intercom or Signal Bell

A small buzzer attached to a long electric cord is pinned or clipped to the bottom sheet near the head of the bed in a place that is easy for the patient to reach. Some units are also equipped with intercoms so that patients and the nurse at the floor desk can speak to each other.

Some types of bedside stands used in nursing homes have built-in, easy-to-operate, push-button panels that control intercom, light switches, and electric bed movement. These are especially useful for patients with limited arm and hand motions.

CLEANING AN OCCUPIED UNIT

The occupied unit is cleaned daily. Most nursing facilities use a cleaning cart set up for this purpose. This saves time and work because the cart is stocked with all the materials and supplies needed.

YOU NEED

    cleaning cart stocked with supplies

YOU DO THIS

Remove any flowers or plants. Trim and add water to fresh flowers. Water and remove dead leaves from plants. (Ask the patient's permission to discard dying flowers.)

Check the unit for unused equipment and return any to its proper storage place.

Check the bedstand cabinet drawer and top for newspapers, food, dishes, medicine cups, used tissues, and paper scraps and remove them. Do not remove newspapers, magazines, or food unless the patient gives permission.

Empty the patient's wastebasket and reline it with a clean bag.

Wash the top of the bedside stand. Wax it, if needed.

Clean the pitcher tray and see that the water glass is clean.

Replace things on the stand.

Refill the patient's supply of tissues, toilet paper, soap, and drinking straws.

Dust the head and foot of the bed and the bedside chair.

Position the unit furniture in order.

Push back the patient's screen curtains.

Adjust the room shades.

Dust any other furniture.

CLEANING THE PATIENT'S BATHROOM

YOU DO THIS

Scrub the sink and tub with cleanser.

Use a toilet brush and disinfectant to scrub the inside of the toilet bowl.

Wash the toilet outside and the entire toilet seat with disinfectant solution.

Be sure toilet paper is on the dispenser and an extra roll nearby.

Wipe the mirror clean.

Be sure the shower curtain is clean.

Be sure other equipment is clean.

Wipe all tiles with disinfectant solution.

Mop the floor with disinfectant solution.

ARRANGING AN OCCUPIED UNIT

Besides the daily cleaning, the unit and room should be checked and arranged several times during the day. A cluttered, untidy room and unit is disturbing to everyone and particularly to a patient. Order makes it easier to find things and gives any patient a sense of security and the feeling that someone cares about him. You will soon learn to run a practiced eye over a room and unit, whenever you enter one, and notice what is out of place or needed. It is important to remember, however, that the geriatric patient is very easily upset by rearrangement of personal belongings. You must adapt your duties to suit the particular wishes of the individual and make every effort to create a cheerful, home-like, and personal atmosphere.

DISINFECTION OF A UNIT

A unit gets a special cleaning, disinfection, and some articles are sterilized several times a year or whenever a patient is discharged from it, when he is transferred to another room of the facility, or if he dies. This disinfection prevents the transfer of germs from one patient to another.

YOU NEED

cleaning cart stocked with supplies

solution of disinfectant in a basin

disposable gloves

YOU DO THIS

Empty the unit of everything but the bed, bedside stand, chair, light, and wastebasket.

Take the rubber drawsheet, washbasin, emesis basin, urinal, and bedpan to the utility room. Clean and sterilize them.

Take the water pitcher, glass, and pitcher tray to the kitchen or service pantry to sterilize them.

Send the blanket to be cleaned or washed.

Place the pillow on the chair.

Fold the mattress in half, head to foot.

Put on the gloves. Wipe every part of the head, legs, and springs of the upper part of the bed with the disinfectant solution.

Lay the mattress flat. Wipe the entire mattress surface, the head and foot ends, and the near side. (Wring the cloth well before using.)

Fold the mattress in half, foot to head.

Wipe the entire foot, legs, and springs of the lower part of the bed.

Pull the underfold of the mattress free until the mattress lies flat. (This turns the mattress foot to head.)

Turn the mattress, under side up. Wipe the flat of the mattress and near side.

Wipe the up surface of the pillow while the pillow is on the chair.

Lay the pillow on the bed, wiped surface down.

Wipe the up side of the pillow.

Wipe all parts of the bedside chair.

Wipe all parts of the inside of the cabinet.

Wipe all parts of the outside of the cabinet.

Wipe the bedside lamp.

Wipe the inside and outside of the wastebasket.

Open windows and close the doors to air the room for several hours.

In some nursing homes the mattress and pillow as well as the bedside equipment are sent to be sterilized in an autoclave. If this is done, they do not need other disinfection.

Most nursing facilities sanitize cabinet equipment in the utility room, and pitchers and water glasses in the kitchen. Both areas have built-in sanitizers operated by valves.

A special sanitizer is used for bedpans only. Bedpans should never be sanitized with other equipment.

Scrub equipment clean and place it in the correct sanitizer. Fill the sanitizer with water and bring it to a boil, then time for 20 minutes.

Wash the rubber or plastic sheet and plastic pillow cover in suds. Rinse, wipe dry on both sides, and then hang over a line to air.

After the equipment is sterilized, return it to the unit.

Put new supplies of tissues, toilet paper, and soap in the bedside stand.

Put a clean bedpan cover and clean bath blanket in the cabinet.

Hang clean towels and washcloth on the stand bar.

Make the bed using clean linen and a clean blanket.

ASEPSIS, OR STERILE TECHNIQUE

Sterile technique and sterile materials are used whenever it is desirable to keep the danger of infection as low as possible. To sterilize means to rid of germs.

In a geriatric facility, sterile materials and techniques are used:

In the examination and in treatment of certain parts of the body, such as the urinary tract.

In the examination and care of skin injuries and operative sites.

When giving injections of any kind.

When taking blood samples or whenever the skin is punctured or opened.

In the collection of any specimens for culture.

The three methods of sterilization in common use are the following:

      Dry heat — an open flame or an oven

      Moist heat — boiling or autoclaving by steam under pressure (Fig. 8)

      Chemicals — antiseptic or germicidal solutions

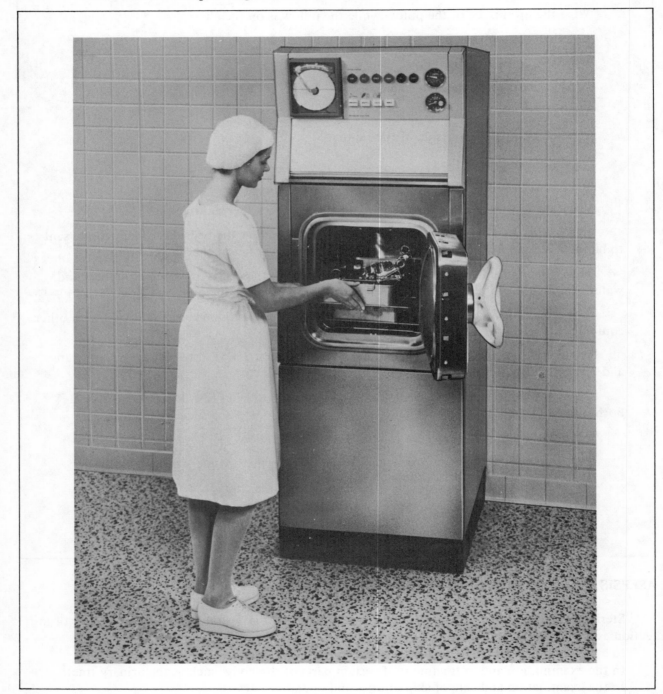

Figure 8. An autoclave for sterilization. (Reprinted by permission of American Sterilizer Co.)

MEETING YOUR GERIATRIC PATIENT'S NEEDS

The amount of time required for sterilization depends on the method used, the size of the article to be sterilized, and extent of exposure to germs.

General Rules for Sterile Techniques

All bundles or containers are labeled before sterilization with the name of the bundle, the size of clothing, the date of sterilization, and the word *sterile*.

Bundles or containers for sterilization are taped shut with *autoclave tape*, which turns color after sterilization and prevents the error of mistaking sterile for unsterile articles.

When opening a sterile package, touch only the outer or unsterile side of the wrapping with your hands.

When removing the lid of a sterile container, touch only the outside of the lid with your hands. Lay the lid down, inside up, and free from contact with unsterilized objects.

The inside of a wrapping or a container is called a sterile field. Nothing unsterile should enter or come near a sterile field. Reaching across a sterile field contaminates it, or makes it unsterile.

Use sterile forceps or sterile gloves to touch any part of, or any object within, a sterile field.

If the wrapping on a sterile bundle becomes wet, the bundle is considered contaminated.

If there is any doubt about the sterility of an article, it should be considered contaminated.

When pouring any antiseptic or sterile solution from a bottle, pour a small amount for discard. Then pour the amount to be used. The solution poured for discard cleans the lip of the container.

When pouring sterile solution from one container to another, do not touch the lips of the containers together.

Many sterile supplies are commercial disposables. Check the label of any package or container for the word *disposable* before discarding any part of it.

Check the wrapper of any disposable sterile package before using. If a wrapper is torn or punctured on a sterile disposable package, the package must not be used, but returned to the company for replacement.

Sterile goods are stored only in areas plainly marked *Sterile Supplies Only*.

All sterile supplies should be checked weekly and unused supplies resterilized.

Putting on Sterile Gloves

YOU DO THIS

Wash your hands.

Check the label on the sterile glove package to be sure you have the right sized gloves.

Open the sterile glove package. Remove the powder packet and powder your hands.

Pick up the first glove by the cuff, touching only the inside of the glove.

Put it on the correct hand without touching any part of the outside.

Pick up the other glove with your gloved hand by slipping your fingers under the cuff.

Work that glove onto your hand, touching only the outside of the glove with your gloved hand.

When you have on both gloves, you must take care to touch only sterile things.

YOUR GERIATRIC PATIENT NEEDS A CLEAN, SAFE, COMFORTABLE PLACE

YOU DO THIS:

Forceps are kept in a container filled with enough antiseptic solution to cover the prongs. The prongs should be in an open position in the solution.

Take hold of the forceps and close them while the prongs are still in solution.

Draw the forceps straight up from the solution without touching the sides or top.

Use the sterile prongs only to handle sterile things. Take care not to touch unsterile objects with them.

Return the forceps to the container during any time when you do not need to handle sterile things.

To replace forceps in their container, close and lower them straight down without touching the sides and top.

Open the prongs after they are in the solution.

SAFETY

Standard Regulations

Every facility is required by law to instruct personnel in state and city building codes and fire and health regulations, such as:
fire and air raid drills
sanitary kitchen and laundry conditions
garbage regulations
Smoking and *No Smoking* areas
adequate facilities for patients and employees
sufficient lighting signs that warn of dangerous areas
keeping doorways, halls, stairways, and exits free of obstacles
the number of people permitted in an elevator at one time
In addition to government regulations, common sense rules should be used anywhere.

Preventing Accidents

Walk, do not run.
Keep to the right side of halls and stairs.
Avoid horseplay.
Take precautions against slipping in any bathroom.
Take precautions against fires.
Avoid overwaxing floors or using scatter rugs.
Pick up or wipe up anything on the floor that does not belong there.
Do not climb on supports that are unsteady or too low to reach high things.

Do not pile things so they can topple over.

Do not leave objects where they are unseen and can be tripped over.

Keep furniture and equipment in repair and good working condition.

Keep equipment neat and orderly to prevent injury from unseen parts.

Check linen for pins or other objects before sending it to the laundry.

Examine the electric cord and plug of any electrical equipment before use. Have frayed cords or loose plugs repaired.

Wheel, do not carry, heavy or awkward equipment.

Keep medicines, cleansers, poisons, and cleaning fluids in a safe place and plainly labeled.

Do not leave filled bottles and containers uncapped.

Be alert for unsafe conditions and do whatever is necessary to correct them.

Special Safety Measures for Geriatric Patients

Special safety precautions are necessary for geriatric patients because they often suffer from conditions such as poor balance, failing vision, and mental confusion that increase the possibilities of accident (Fig. 9).

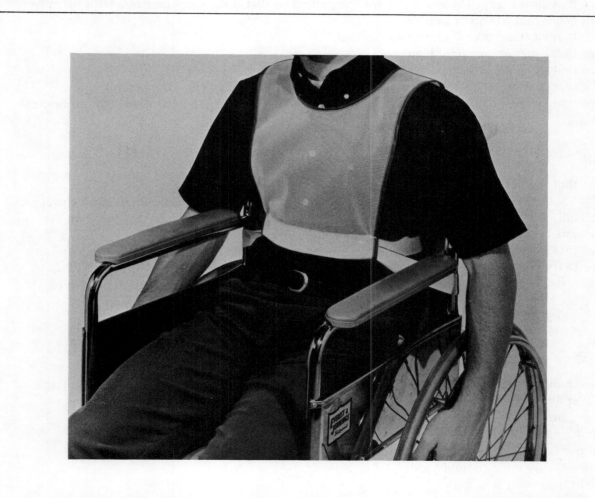

Figure 9. A chest restraint for a wheelchair patient that prevents him from sliding or falling from the chair. (Reprinted by permission of © J. T. Posey Co.)

Here are some special precautions.

For Bed

Use bed rails when a patient is sleeping or confused.

Do not allow a patient to get out of a high bed without help.

Do not use hot water bottles or heating pads without a doctor's order. A hot water bottle should be filled with warm water — never hot water.

Do not allow a patient to smoke in bed.

Wipe the bed and mattress often with a mild antiseptic.

Keep the bed clothing clean, orderly, and dry.

Keep the patient's belongings within easy reach so that he will not have to stretch to reach them.

For bed support, use rolled bath blankets, sheets, or towels rather than pillows, which might cover the face and interfere with breathing.

For Clothing and Walking Equipment

See that clothing is the correct size for the patient so that it does not interfere with his movements or cause him to trip or fumble.

See that clothing is kept clean and mended.

See that shoes are repaired regularly.

See that the patient wears clothes suitable to the weather.

See that clothing is lightweight and does not drag on the floor or tire the patient.

See that walking equipment is kept in good condition and that the patient uses the equipment correctly.

For Bath

See that the patient uses an electric shaver rather than a safety razor.

Make sure that the patient uses grab rails on tub and toilet. Never let a patient use a towel rack as a grab rail.

Be alert for and clean floors wet with water, urine, or other fluid.

See that the room is warm and draft-free while the patient is bathing.

See that the room is well lighted.

Never use bath water hotter than 105°F. (The geriatric patient's skin is more sensitive to temperature changes than is the younger adult, and he can be burned more easily.)

Use nonslip tape or a nonslip suction pad in the tub.

For Food

Never allow a patient to use a sharp knife or other utensil with which he can injure himself.

Use spillproof dishes and glasses.

Use unbreakable dishes and glassware.

Wash and sterilize all dishes and glassware after use.

Prepare special diets exactly as ordered.

Use a sturdy table to hold food.

Light the eating area well.

For Room

Cover radiators.
Use nonslip floor covering.
Have doors open in against walls.
Use crossbars over windows with low sills.
Use sturdy, nontippable furniture (Fig. 10).

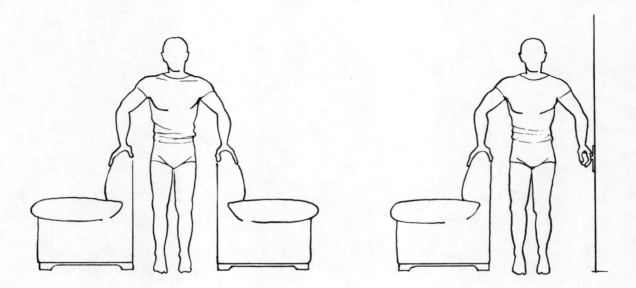

Figure 10. Left: *A patient using sturdy chairs for support when standing.* Right: *A patient using a sturdy chair and a door for support when standing. (Reprinted from* Elementary Rehabilitation Nursing Care, *U.S. Public Health Service, Division of Nursing.)*

For Hallways and Stairs

See that these areas are well-lighted throughout.
Have handrails on both sides of stairs.
Have beginning and ends of rails shaped differently than the center portion so they can be identified by touch as well as sight.
Paint with white or yellow the first and last step of a series of steps.
Use nonslip floor covering.
Block stairway with gate.

4

YOUR GERIATRIC PATIENT NEEDS TO BE ADMITTED, TRANSFERRED, OR DISCHARGED FROM A NURSING HOME

STUDY GUIDE

How is a patient admitted to a geriatric nursing home?

Is admission temporary or permanent?

What does a person who is entering a nursing home need?

How are these needs met by a nursing home?

How does a new admission patient feel?

How can you help to make him feel at ease?

What is a "buddy" or "sister" system?

Tell how to prepare for an admission patient.

What is a check sheet for admission?

Tell what you do during admission of a new patient.

What should you do with all the new patient's belongings?

How do you orient the patient to his program?

Why might a patient be transferred from one level of nursing care to another?

What must be done when a patient is discharged?

ADMISSION to a geriatric nursing home may be on a voluntary basis, through the recommendation of a doctor, or through social service workers. Acceptance in a nursing home is determined by the patient's needs, the space available, and the patient's ability to pay for the services offered.

Admission may be temporary or permanent, depending on the patient's needs. A stroke patient may require only a month or two of a learning program in activities of daily living (ADL) that enables him to return to his own home. Another patient with a number of chronic diseases, which indicate a need for increasing amounts of medical supervision and care, might be admitted on a permanent basis.

Whether as a temporary or permanent resident, any person enters a nursing home as though he were moving to a new life. He needs to orient himself, to maintain contact with his old life, and to establish his new home as his own.

When possible, a prospective permanent resident is allowed to visit the nursing home for a week or two on several occasions before his final move. Any patient who is able should be permitted to visit his old home whenever such a visit is convenient for him, his family, or friends. He should also be allowed visitors as often as they care to come. On entering a nursing home, the patient should be encouraged to bring small personal items, such as a picture or books, which mark his room or unit as belonging to him.

Even so, anyone who is admitted to any nursing facility is nervous and insecure. It is your job to lessen his fears and to help him feel at ease as quickly as possible. Be friendly and cheerful. Show consideration for his feelings and wishes. Explain the daily routine of the nursing level to which he is admitted.

Many nursing homes use a "buddy" or "sister" system to help the newcomer. This means that a long-standing resident of the same sex is asked to be with the newcomer as often as possible for the first week or so after his arrival. The long-standing resident may be a roommate or nearby neighbor and is someone who is able to show the newcomer about the nursing home and answer some of the many anxious questions that trouble him until he knows his way.

Many nursing homes have traditional ways of welcoming the newcomer. These range from special greetings from each member of the staff or newcomer parties to welcoming gifts, such as a plant or handy personal item that was made in the nursing home's occupational therapy room.

PREPARING FOR AN ADMISSION

Go to the room. If there are other patients in the room, tell them a new patient is coming.
Check the bed, bedside stand, clothes dresser, and closet. See that they are clean and ready for use.
Put a new box of tissues at the bedside.

CHECK SHEET FOR AN ADMISSION

Because there are always so many things to do for a new admission and because these things vary from one facility to another, admission check sheets are commonly used. Such a sheet lists all the admission requirements for a particular level of nursing care.

You follow the list, as you admit the patient, and check off with a pen each thing you do.

DURING ADMISSION

Introduce yourself to the patient.
Greet him by his last name (*Example:* Mr. Smith.) as you would a welcome guest.
Take the patient to his room. If he is with a family member or friend, invite that person to accompany you to the room.
In the room, introduce the patient to his "buddy" and to any other patients.
Show the patient his unit. Tell about and show everything that will belong to him. Explain anything unusual, such as the signal light.
Show the patient his toilet and inquire if he would like to use it.
Help the patient to unpack and put his belongings in his drawers and closets. (Most nursing homes have systems for marking the clothing belonging to a patient.)
Label any personal articles, such as a wheelchair or cane, with the patient's name and room number.

Give the patient written instructions about the times and places for meals and occupational, physical, and recreational activities. Go over this program with him, explaining anything he does not understand.

If the charge nurse okays it, see that he has fresh water and a drinking glass at his bedside.

TRANSFERRING A PATIENT

Sometimes a patient is transferred from one level of nursing care to another, in a different part of the building. A very sick person might be transferred to a facility for acutely ill patients. Someone might be removed from a room with other patients and be put in isolation. Such transfers are temporary and the patient retains his permanent room, returning to it when he recovers. Arrangements for permanent transfer are made through the Main Office.

PERMANENT TRANSFER

YOU DO THIS

Explain to the patient that he is being transferred. The charge nurse should tell him why.

Be sure the unit to which he is going is prepared to receive him.

Collect all the patient's effects and take them with him. If he has clothing stored, the clothing book or sheet must be taken and the clothes signed for at the new area. His chart and desk records, medications and other items must also be taken. A transfer slip is made out and must be signed by the receiving nurse. Be sure the chart is up to date before taking it. The last entry on the nurse's notes should be the time of transfer and "Patient transferred to _____."

A stretcher or wheelchair and sometimes the patient's bed may be used in the transfer. The choice would depend on the patient's condition and where he is going. Follow the rules for stretcher or wheelchair use.

When you and the patient reach the new area, introduce the patient to the nurse in charge. Have her sign the transfer slip and clothes sheet.

Take the charge nurse aside and give her a brief oral report on the patient. Do not let the patient hear you.

Give the nurse the patient's belongings and records.

Stay with the patient until he is settled into his new unit.

Return to your station and see that the vacated unit is cleaned to receive a new patient.

5

YOUR GERIATRIC PATIENT NEEDS PHYSICAL THERAPY

STUDY GUIDE

What causes the slowing down of body function in the aged?

How can these changes be delayed and sometimes avoided?

What is physical therapy?

Tell four aims of physical therapy.

How does a doctor determine specific physical therapy for a patient?

Tell four things that can be included in a patient's program of physical therapy.

Body Joints

On what does the normal extent of motion in a human body depend?

What is a joint?

What is a gliding joint? Give an example.

What is a hinge joint? Give an example.

What is a condyloid joint? Give an example.

What is a ball-and-socket joint? Give an example.

What is a pivot joint? Give an example.

Body Motion

Tell why body motion is important to the health of any person.

How does the average person perform body motion?

Why is planned activity important for an aged person?

Who prescribes exercises for an aged person?

Range of Motion Exercises (R.O.M.)

What name is given to prescribed exercises?

What is the abbreviation for that name?

What does range of motion mean?

What is the difference between normal range of motion and functional range of motion?

What are activities of daily living?

Tell the four kinds of range of motion exercises?

How do free active R.O.M. exercises differ from passive R.O.M. exercises?

How do resistive R.O.M. exercises differ from active assistive R.O.M. exercises?

Under what conditions are range of motion exercises most effective.

Tell what you should do for a patient before, during, and after R.O.M. exercises.

Normal Body Motions

What is neutral position?

In which three ways can a person assume neutral position while lying down?

What is a midline and how is it used?

What is flexion?

What is extension?

What is hyperextension?

What is abduction?

What is adduction?

What is rotation?

THE PHYSICAL THERAPY PROGRAM

Any aging person can expect progressive slowing down and breaking down of body functioning. These are the results of disease, injury, time, and neglect. With proper treatment, however, such changes can be delayed and sometimes avoided; a patient can be rehabilitated or trained to function despite a disability. Physical therapy is the name for this treatment.

Physical therapy is treatment through stimulation of the body or a body part. The aims of physical therapy are:

To maintain and increase normal body function.
To prevent loss of function when possible.
To train a patient to substitute functioning when loss occurs.
To help a patient become as independent as possible.

Specific physical therapy for the individual patient is ordered by the doctor after testing and evaluation. A patient's program usually includes more than one of the following:

Range of motion exercises

Activities of daily living

Use of special equipment, such as Hubbard Tank, Whirlpool, ultrasound, or hot wax tank

Occupational therapy

BODY JOINTS

The normal extent of motion in a human depends on the ways in which 206 bones are joined to form the body skeleton. When one bone connects to another so that a part of the body is movable, the bone connection is called a joint.

Here are some main kinds of joints:

Condyloid joint. Two bones connect to allow angle movement in two directions. (*Example:* wrists.)

Ball-and-socket joint. Two bones connect to allow movement in all directions. (*Example:* shoulders and hips.)

Gliding joint. Two bones connect by sliding against each other. (*Example:* small bones of the wrists and ankles.)

Hinge joint. Two bones connect to allow angle movement in one direction. (*Example:* elbows and knees.)

Pivot joint. Two bones connect to allow one to rotate around part of the other. (*Example:* spinal bones.)

BODY MOTION

Activity or body motion is important to the health of any individual of any age. Motion increases blood circulation and this improves the functioning of all body parts, in particular the cardiovascular and respiratory systems. Motion also:

Helps maintain the range of movement in body joints.

Prevents deformities by keeping joints moving freely.

Increases the range of joint movement in people with decreased range of movement.

Helps maintain muscle strength.

Increases muscle strength after loss of strength following sickness or injury.

Helps maintain good coordination of the nervous system.

Aids all healing, helps prevent swelling of the legs and feet, and helps prevent decubitus ulcers from forming.

Increases a person's endurance (the ability to perform the same movement over and over during a length of time).

A younger person makes enough natural motions in his routine of daily life to keep his body in function. He also seeks exercise, such as swimming, playing tennis, and dancing.

Aging causes a gradual slowing of all body activities. Unless a plan of activity is carried out, a geriatric person loses more and more of his ability to perform full motions. A plan of activity can mean the difference between a patient becoming a helpless invalid and being able to care for himself.

The plan of activity is ordered by the doctor to suit the patient's individual need. It may vary from a daily walk to special exercises for different parts of the patient's body.

Special exercises needed by the patient are determined by testing the extent of movement in his joints and the extent of self-care he can perform. These special exercises are called range of motion (R.O.M.) exercises.

RANGE OF MOTION (R.O.M.)

Range of motion (R.O.M.) means the full extent of movement in a body joint.

Normal range of motion means the ability to perform a full movement of a body joint.

Functional range of motion means a less than normal ability to move a body joint but enough ability to allow a person to perform activities of daily living.

Activities of daily living (A.D.L.) are movements made in the course of daily self-care.

Part of a sample R.O.M. test is shown in Figure 11. It is used to determine the extent of R.O.M. in a patient. Based on the results of this test, a doctor can prescribe specific exercises to suit the patient's individual needs. The patient is retested regularly and his exercise program adjusted to suit his changing needs.

Kinds of Range of Motion (R.O.M.) Exercises

Free active R.O.M. exercises are done entirely by the patient.

Resistive R.O.M. exercises are done by a patient against pull provided by another person, a weight, or a machine.

Active assistive R.O.M. exercises are done in part by the patient and in part by another person or a machine.

Passive R.O.M. exercises are done to a patient by another person or machine without any help from the patient.

A prescription for R.O.M. exercises on a particular patient may require the use of one or more kinds of motion exercises.

Example: A patient may need free active R.O.M. exercises for his shoulders, resistive R.O.M. exercises for one arm, and passive R.O.M. for both legs.

Using Range of Motion Exercises

Range of motion exercises are most effective when done at regular, frequent intervals, and when one motion is repeated a limited number of times. (For example, it is better to do an R.O.M. exercise twice a day for five times at each exercise period than once a day for ten times.)

Figure 11. Sample range of motion test sheet. (By permission of New York University Medical Center, Department of Rehabilitative Medicine.)

NAME _____ AGE _____

DISABILITY _____ DIAGNOSIS _____ IN ____ OUT ____

RANGE OF MOTION TEST FOR UPPER EXTREMITY

1. Anatomical position is starting position. Range is measured with cauda as 0°, cranium as 180°. Rotating motions are from the midsagittal plane as 0° to lateral plane as 180°.

2. All ranges are expressed as passive range of motion. Check muscle chart attached for limitations caused by tightness, weakness, spasm, or contracture.

3. The scale is divided into units of 10°. Range of motion is recorded by filling in area of range directly on attached sketch with date and examiner's initial.

4. Use of same sheet for subsequent tests is recorded in same color and dated accordingly.

5. Retrogression is marked by diagonal lines over area of previous test and dated.

6. If position is other than in sketch, indicate S for supine, P for prone.

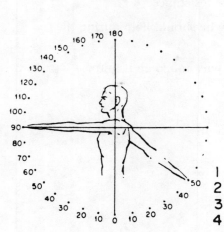

Shoulder

Flexion	0- 90
Flexion and rotation of scapula	90-180
Extension and rotation of scapula	180-90
Extension	90- -50

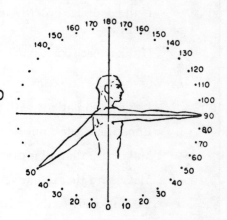

Limitations

	L		R	
	Fl.	Ext.	Fl.	Ext.
1				
2				
3				
4				

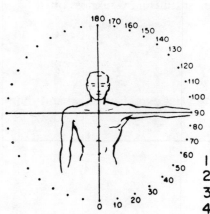

Shoulder

Abduction	0- 90
Abduction and rotation of scapula	90-180
Adduction and rotation of scapula	180-90
Adduction	90- 0

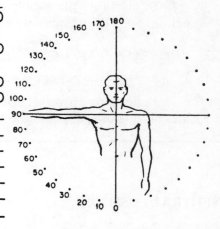

Limitations

	L		R	
	Abd.	Add.	Abd.	Add.
1				
2				
3				
4				

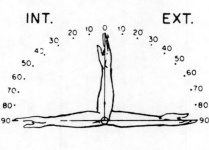

INT.　　　　　EXT.

Shoulder Rotation

Elbow flexed	90°
External rotation	0- 90
Internal rotation	0- 90

EXT.　　　　　INT.

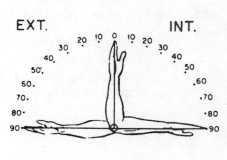

Limitations

	L		R	
	Int.	Ext.	Int.	Ext.
1				
2				
3				
4				

YOU DO THIS

Before R.O.M. Exercises

Dress the patient so that he can move freely and without embarrassment.

Get the full attention and cooperation of the patient. Put him at ease.

Before each new exercise, describe the exercise to the patient. Tell the patient in what ways the exercise should affect and help him. Tell the patient how he should feel while the exercise is being done. Tell him what he should do during the exercise.

If the exercise is *free active*, tell the patient to perform it alone.

If the exercise is *resistive*, tell the patient to pull against the resistance.

If the exercise is *active assistive*, explain to the patient how he should help during the movement.

If the exercise is *passive*, tell the patient to relax the body part and keep it limp.

During R.O.M. Exercises

Inspire the patient with confidence in your ability to exercise him.

Encourage self-confidence in the patient.

Make sure that all movements are as complete as possible.

Make sure that all movements are smooth and steady.

Do not overtire the patient.

Do not cause unnecessary pain.

Be alert for unfavorable changes in the patient, such as pain or unusual weakness or pallor. Stop the exercise session if any of these occurs.

After R.O.M. Exercises

See that the patient is comfortable.

Report any changes noticed in the patient either between the last exercise period and the present one or changes in the patient during the treatment.

NEUTRAL POSITION

Standing or lying straight with heels together and arms at the sides with palms toward the body is called the neutral position (Fig. 12).

This position can be assumed in the following lying positions:
    Lateral: lying on one side.
    Prone: lying on the abdomen and face.
    Supine: lying on the back.

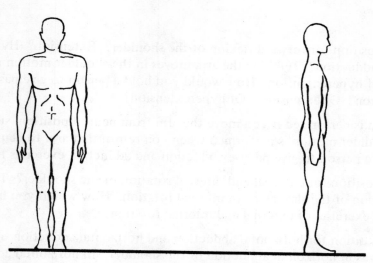

Figure 12. Neutral position. (Reprinted from Elementary Rehabilitation Nursing Care, *U.S. Public Health Service, Division of Nursing.)*

A midline is an imaginary line, dividing the body or a part of the body lengthwise into two equal halves. It is used as a reference when describing or performing body motions.

The following words are used to describe body motions:

Flexion: bending. *looking down*
Extension: straightening. *looking up*
Hyperextension: carrying a straightened movement beyond neutral position.
Abduction: moving the part away from the midline.
Adduction: moving the part toward the midline.
Rotation: turning a limb or body part.

STUDY GUIDE

Head and Neck Motions

What is the starting position for all head and neck R.O.M. exercises?

In what position is a person when he bends his neck to look upward? To look downward?

In what position is a person when he bends his head toward his right shoulder? In what position is a person when he bends his head toward his left shoulder?

In what position is a person when he turns his head to look over his right shoulder? In what position is a person when he turns his head to look over his left shoulder?

How would you hold a patient to give all passive R.O.M. head and neck exercises?

Body Trunk Motions

What is the starting position for all body trunk exercises?

How does the trunk move during flexion? During extension? During hyperextension?

In what position is a person whose trunk is bent sideways to the right? To the left?

In what position is a person whose trunk and shoulders are turned to the right while his hips remain in neutral position? Whose trunk and shoulders are turned to the left? Whose trunk and shoulders are in neutral position but whose hips are turned to the right? To the left?

How would you hold a person to give all passive R.O.M. exercises to the body trunk?

Shoulder Motions

What is the starting position for forward flexion of the shoulder? Extension? Hyperextension? Abduction and adduction? Tell how the arm moves in the shoulder motion of forward flexion. Of extension. Of hyperextension. How would you hold a person to give passive R.O.M. shoulder exercises of flexion? Of extension? Of hyperextension?

What shoulder motion is performed if you move the arm from neutral position, sideways, to over the head? What shoulder motion is performed when you return that arm to neutral position? How would you hold a person to give passive abduction and adduction exercises to the shoulder?

What is the starting position for external and internal rotation of the shoulder? Tell how an arm moves in external rotation of the shoulder. In internal rotation. How would you hold a person to give passive shoulder exercises of external and internal rotation?

What is the starting position for horizontal abduction and horizontal adduction of the shoulder? Tell how an arm moves in horizontal abduction of the shoulder. In horizontal adduction. How would you hold a person to give passive R.O.M. exercises of horizontal abduction and horizontal adduction to his shoulder?

What is the starting position for elevation and depression of the shoulder? Tell how the shoulder moves in elevation. In depression. How would you hold a person to give passive R.O.M. exercises of elevation and depression of the shoulder?

What is the starting position for protraction and retraction of the shoulder? Tell how the arm and shoulder move in protraction. In retraction. How would you hold a person to give passive R.O.M. exercises of protraction and retraction to his shoulder?

Elbow Motions

What is the starting position for flexion and extension of the elbow? Tell how the arm moves in flexion and extension of the elbow. How would you hold a person to give passive R.O.M. exercises of flexion and extension to his elbow?

Forearm Motions

What is the starting position for pronation and supination of the forearm? What is the name of the forearm motion performed when the palm turns downward? What is supination? How would you hold a person to give passive R.O.M. exercises of pronation and supination?

Wrist Motions

What is the starting position for flexion, extension, and hyperextension of the wrist? How is the wrist moved in flexion? In extension? In hyperextension? How would you hold a person to give passive wrist exercises?

Finger Motions

What is the starting position for flexion and extension of the finger? What motion is performed by making a fist? By opening the hand? How would you hold a person to give passive R.O.M. finger exercises of flexion and extension?

What is the starting position for abduction and adduction of the fingers? Tell how the fingers move in abduction. In adduction. How would you hold a person to give passive R.O.M. finger exercises of abduction and adduction?

Thumb Motions

What is the starting position for flexion and extension of the thumb? In what position is a person's thumb when it is in flexion? In extension?

What is the starting position for abduction and adduction of the thumb? In what position is the thumb during abduction? During adduction?

What is the starting position for opposition of the thumb? In what position is the thumb during opposition?

How would you hold a person to give all passive R.O.M. exercises to his thumb?

Hip Motions

What is the starting position for all hip motions? Tell how the leg moves in hip flexion. In hip extension. In hip hyperextension. How would you hold a person to give passive R.O.M. exercises of flexion and extension to his hip? Of hyperextension?

What motion is performed when a leg and its toes are turned inward? When they are turned outward? How would you hold a person to give passive R.O.M. exercises of internal and external rotation of the hip?

Tell how the leg moves in abduction and adduction of the hip. How would you hold a person to give passive R.O.M. exercises of abduction and adduction of his hip?

Knee Motions

What is the starting position for knee motion? In what position is a person's knee when it is in flexion? In extension? Tell two ways in which you could hold a person to give passive R.O.M. exercises of flexion and extension of the knee.

Ankle Motions

What is the starting position for all ankle motions? Tell how the foot and toes move when the ankle is in dorsal flexion. In plantar flexion. How would you hold a person to give passive R.O.M. exercises of dorsal and plantar flexion of the ankle?

Tell how the foot and toes move when the ankle is in eversion. In inversion. How would you hold a person to give passive R.O.M. exercises of eversion and inversion to his ankle?

Toe Motions

What is the starting position for all toe motions?

In what position are a person's toes during flexion? During extension? How would you hold a person to give passive R.O.M. exercises of flexion and extension of the toes?

In what position are a person's toes when they are spread apart? In what position are a person's toes when they return to neutral position after being spread? How would you hold a person to give passive R.O.M. exercises of abduction and adduction of the toes?

THE THREE GROUPS OF HEAD AND NECK MOTIONS[*]

1. START with head in neutral position.

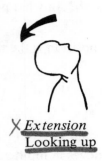

Extension
Looking up

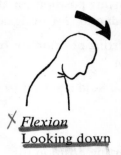

Flexion
Looking down

2. START with head in neutral position.

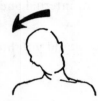

Right Lateral Flexion
Bending head toward right shoulder

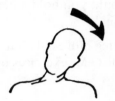

Left Lateral Flexion
Bending head toward left shoulder

3. START with head in neutral position.

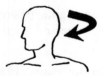

Right Rotation
Turning head to right to see over shoulder

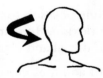

Left Rotation
Turning head to left to see over shoulder

Hold for All Passive Head and Neck Motions

Cup your hands over the patient's ears and grasp the head in a firm hold.

---

[*]All illustrations for range of motion exercises on pages 68–79 are from *Elementary Rehabilitative Nursing Care,* U.S. Public Health Service, Division of Nursing.

THE THREE GROUPS OF BODY TRUNK MOTIONS

1. START with body in neutral position.

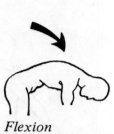 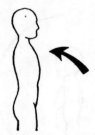 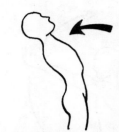

Flexion
Bending forward

Extension
Straightening

Hyperextension
Moving body backward
from the waist

2. START with body in neutral position.

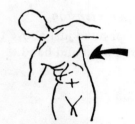 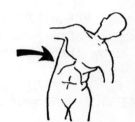

Right Lateral Flexion
Bending sideways to right

Left Lateral Flexion
Bending sideways to left

3. START with body in neutral position.
   while keeping hips in neutral position

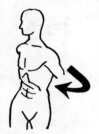 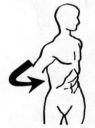

Right Rotation
Turning shoulders to right

Left Rotation
Turning shoulders to left

Alternative: Turn hips to left or right while keeping shoulders in neutral position

Hold for All Passive Body Trunk Motions
Reach around the patient's back to grasp his far shoulder with one of your hands,
allowing the patient's head to rest on your forearm. Grasp the patient's near shoulder
with your other hand. As an alternative, hold both the patient's legs at the knees with one or both
of your hands, while the patient rotates his trunk.

THE SIX GROUPS OF SHOULDER MOTIONS

1. START with arm in neutral position.

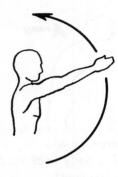 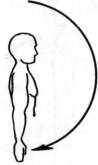 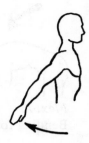

Forward Flexion
Moving arm forward
and upward

Extension
Returning arm to
neutral position

Hyperextension
Moving arm backward
from neutral position

Hold for Passive Flexion, Extension, and Hyperextension
Stand facing the side of the patient to be exercised. Place your near hand just above the patient's elbow. Use your other hand to support the patient's wrist and hand.

2. START with arm in neutral position.

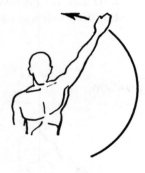 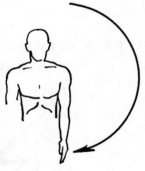

Abduction
Moving arm sideways, away from
the body and over the head

Adduction
Returning arm to neutral position

Hold for Passive Abduction and Adduction
Stand facing the front or back of the patient. Grasp the patient's arm just above the elbow.
Use your other hand to support the patient's wrist and hand.

3. START with arm at shoulder height and elbow bent at a right angle.

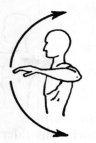

External Rotation
Turning the upper part of the arm so
that the forearm and palm face forward

Internal Rotation
Turning the upper part of the arm so
that the forearm and palm face backward

Hold for Passive Internal and External Rotation
With patient on his back, face the arm to be exercised. With one hand, grasp the patient's arm just below the elbow. Use your other hand to support the patient's wrist and hand.

4. START with arm at shoulder height and elbow straight.

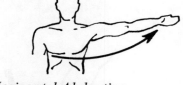

Horizontal Abduction
Moving arm back as far as possible

Horizontal Adduction
Moving arm forward and across the chest

Hold for Passive Horizontal Abduction and Adduction
Stand facing patient's head on side to be exercised. Grasp the patient's arm just above the elbow. Use your other hand to support the patient's wrist and hand.

5. START with arm in neutral position.

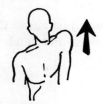

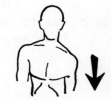

Elevation
Lifting shoulder

Depression
Lowering shoulder

Hold for Passive Elevation and Depression
Stand facing patient's head on side to be exercised. Grasp the patient's arm just above the elbow. Use your other hand to support the patient's hand and wrist.

6. START with arm at shoulder height in forward flexion.

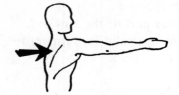

Protraction
Reaching forward as far as possible

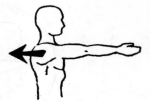

Retraction
Drawing shoulder and arm back from
protraction position

Hold for Passive Protraction and Retraction
Stand facing patient's side to be exercised. Grasp the patient's arm just above the elbow.
Use your other hand to support the patient's hand and wrist.

THE ONE GROUP OF ELBOW MOTIONS

START with arm in neutral position.

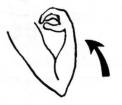

Flexion
Bending elbow and bringing forearm
and hand toward shoulder

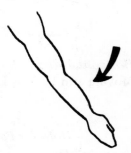

Extension
Returning forearm and hand to neutral position

Hold for Passive Flexion and Extension
Stand facing the arm to be exercised. Grasp the patient's arm just above the elbow.
Use your other hand to support the patient's wrist and hand.

THE ONE GROUP OF FOREARM MOTIONS

START with elbow at waist, bent at a right angle, with palm facing body.

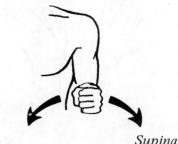

Pronation
Turning palm downward

Supination
Turning palm upward

Hold for Passive Pronation and Supination
Use both your hands to grasp the patient's hand and wrist.

THE TWO GROUPS OF WRIST MOTIONS

1. START with hand in extension, palm upward.

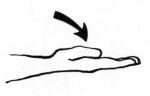

Flexion
Bending wrist so that palm
faces forearm

Extension
Returning hand to
starting position

Hyperextension
Moving hand so that the back of
it faces forearm

2. START with hand in extension.

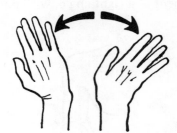

Radial Deviation
Moving hand sideways so that
thumb is toward forearm

Ulnar Deviation
Moving hand sideways so that little
finger is toward forearm

Hold for all Passive Wrist Motions
Use one of your hands to grasp the patient's arm just above the wrist.
Use your other hand to hold the patient's hand.

THE TWO GROUPS OF FINGER MOTIONS

1. START with hand in extension.

Flexion
Making a fist

Extension
Opening hand

Hold for Passive Flexion and Extension
Use one of your hands to support the patient's forearm and wrist.
Use the fingers on your other hand to open and close the patient's fingers.

2. START with hand in extension.

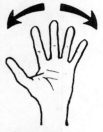

Abduction
Spreading fingers

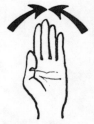

Adduction
Closing fingers

Hold for Passive Abduction and Adduction
Use both of your hands to hold the fingers of one of the patient's hands.

THE THREE GROUPS OF THUMB MOTIONS

1. START with thumb in extension.

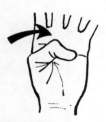

Flexion
Bending all joints

Extension
Straightening all joints

2. START with hand, palm upward, in extension.

Abduction
Raising thumb

Adduction
Returning thumb

3. START with hand in extension.

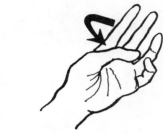

Opposition
Touching tips of thumb and little finger

Hold for all Passive Thumb Motions
Support the patient's hand and fingers with one of your hands.
Use your other hand to hold the patient's thumb.

THE THREE GROUPS OF HIP MOTIONS

1. START with leg in neutral position.

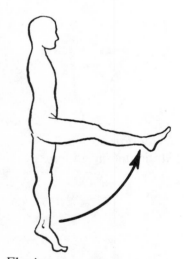 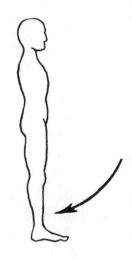 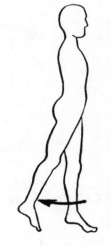

Flexion	*Extension*	*Hyperextension*
Moving leg forward from hip	Returning leg to neutral position	Moving leg back from hip

Hold for Passive Flexion and Extension
Support the patient's leg by placing his ankle on your upper arm or shoulder.
Place your hand over his knee to keep it straight.
Hold for Passive Hyperextension
Turn patient on his abdomen. Place one of your hands under patient's ankle and grasp it.
Place your other hand just above his knee.

2. START with legs in neutral position.

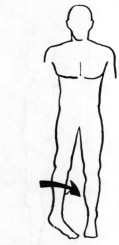 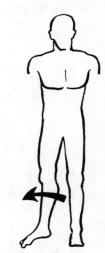

Internal Rotation
Turning leg and toes inward

External Rotation
Turning leg and toes outward

Hold for Passive Internal and External Rotation
Stand facing side to be exercised. Grasp the patient's ankle with one hand.
Place your other hand on top of his knee.

3. START with leg in neutral position.

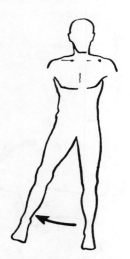 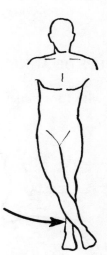

Abduction
Moving one leg outward

Adduction
Returning leg to neutral position and
crossing it over the other leg

Hold for Passive Abduction and Adduction
Stand facing the side to be exercised. Place one hand just above the knee.
Use your other hand to support the ankle.

THE ONE GROUP OF KNEE MOTIONS

START with leg in neutral position.

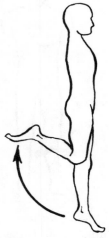 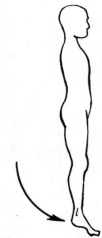

Flexion
Bending knee and moving foot
toward back of leg

Extension
Returning leg to neutral position

Hold for Passive Flexion and Extension
With patient on his back, put hip in flexion and bend knee. Place one hand under leg
just above the knee for support. Use your other hand to grasp the ankle from beneath.
With patient on his abdomen, place one hand on back of leg just above knee.
Use your other hand to grasp the ankle from beneath.

THE TWO GROUPS OF ANKLE MOTIONS

1. START with foot in neutral position.

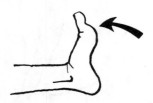 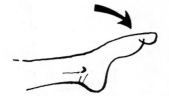

Dorsal Flexion
Moving foot and toes toward the shin

Plantar Flexion
Moving foot and toes toward the heel

Hold for Passive Flexion and Extension
Place one hand on the patient's knee to prevent flexion. With your other hand,
hold the patient's foot so that the heel rests in your palm and the sole rests against your forearm.

2. START with foot in neutral position.

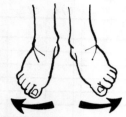 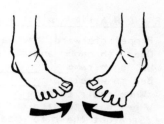

Eversion
Turning foot and toes outward

Inversion
Turning foot and toes inward

Hold for Passive Eversion and Inversion
Use one of your hands to hold the patient's heel.
Use the other hand to grasp the top of the foot.

THE TWO GROUPS OF TOE MOTIONS

1. START with foot in neutral position.

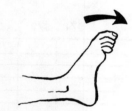 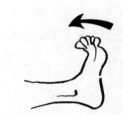

Flexion
Bending toes toward sole

Extension
Bending toes toward shin

Hold for Passive Flexion and Extension
Hold patient's foot with one hand. Use your other hand to move the toes.

2. START with foot in neutral position.

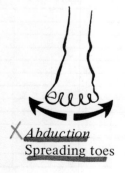 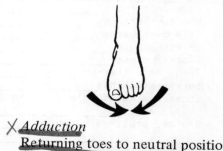

Abduction
Spreading toes

Adduction
Returning toes to neutral position

Hold for Passive Abduction and Adduction
Use both hands to grasp patient's toes.

WHEELCHAIR ACTIVITIES

	G/1	G/2	Date	I
Propel: forward, backward, turn				
Open, through, and close door				
Up, down ramp				
Bed to wheelchair				
Wheelchair to bed				
Wheelchair to straight chair				
Straight chair to wheelchair				
Wheelchair to easy chair, couch				
Easy chair, couch to wheelchair				
Wheelchair to toilet (high toilet seat, regular seat)				
Toilet to wheelchair				
Adjust clothing				
Wheelchair to tub				
Tub to wheelchair				
Wheelchair to shower (chair in stall shower, or tub)				
Shower to wheelchair				
TRAVEL: Wheelchair to car - on curb				
Car to wheelchair - on curb				
Wheelchair to car - no curb				
Car to wheelchair - no curb				
Place wheelchair in car - on street				

SELFCARE ACTIVITIES

HYGIENE (TOILET ACTIVITIES)

	G/1	G/2	Date	I
Comb, brush hair				
Brush teeth				
Shave (electric razor, safety razor), put on make up				
Turn faucet				
Wash, dry hands and face				
Wash, dry body and extremities				
Take bath (wheelchair, walking)				
Take shower (wheelchair, walking)				
Use urinal, bedpan				

EATING ACTIVITIES

	G/1	G/2	Date	I
Eat with spoon				
Eat with fork				
Cut meat				
Handle: straw, cup, glass				

DRESSING ACTIVITIES

	G/1	G/2	Date	I
Undershirt--bra				
Shorts--panties				
Slip-over garment				
Shirt--blouse				
Slacks--dress				
Tying neck tie--bow				
Socks--stockings				
Shoes (laces, buckles, slip-on)				
Coat, jacket				
Braces, prosthesis, corset				

MISCELLANEOUS HAND-ACTIVITIES	G/1	G/2	Date	I
Write name and address				
Manage: watch				
match or cigarette lighter				
cigarette				
book, newspaper				
handkerchief				
lights; chain, switch, knob				
telephone: receiver, dial, coins				
handle: purse, coins, paper money				

WALKING ACTIVITIES	G/1	G/2	Date	I
Open, go through, and close door				
Walking outside				
Walking carrying				

STANDING UP AND SITTING DOWN	G/1	G/2	Date	I
Up from wheelchair				
Down on wheelchair				
Up from bed				
Down on bed				
Up from straight chair				
Down on straight chair				
Up from straight chair at table				
Down on straight chair at table				
Up from easy chair				
Down on easy chair				
Up from center of couch				
Down on center of couch				
Up from toilet				
Down on toilet				
Adjust clothing				
Into car, on curb, up curb				
Out of car				
Down on floor				
Up from floor				

CLIMBING AND TRAVELING ACTIVITIES	G/1	G/2	Date	I
Up flight of stairs (railing, no railing)				
Down flight of stairs (railing, no railing)				
Into and out of car, taxi				
Walk one block and back				
Down curb, cross street, on curb				
Into bus				
Sit down, get up from bus seat				
Out of bus				

Figures 13 and 14. Parts of an A.D.L. test. (By permission of Edith Lawton and New York University Medical Center, Department of Rehabilitative Medicine.)

STUDY GUIDE

Activities of Daily Living

What motions of self-care are included in A.D.L.?

How is an A.D.L. program designed?

What three things should you understand about any A.D.L. program?

Tell eight ways in which you can help a patient with his A.D.L. program.

How are A.D.L. goals influenced by the individual patient?

Name some adaptive things used in A.D.L. for moving about in bed, personal grooming, dressing and undressing, eating, using hands, and using the toilet.

How does occupational therapy help a patient?

What forms of recreational therapy are also good physical therapy?

ACTIVITIES OF DAILY LIVING (A.D.L.)

Activities of daily living are motions of self-care that are learned by the child and become habit with the adult. They include:

> moving about in bed
> personal grooming
> dressing and undressing
> eating
> using the hands
> walking
> using the toilet

Many health conditions of the geriatric patient can affect his ability to do these things. Nursing personnel, assigned to the everyday care of a patient, should know about the patient's health and should be alert to recognize changes in his ability to care for himself.

A.D.L. Tests

A geriatric patient is given regular A.D.L. tests to determine limitations and changes in his abilities to perform self-care (Figs. 13 and 14). After each test, a specific A.D.L. program is designed for the individual patient, who needs reminding, remotivating, or retraining to help him perform self-care activities to the best of his ability. Such an A.D.L. program cannot succeed unless the nursing personnel assigned to the patient work with the patient and with the A.D.L. nurse.

Your Role in A.D.L.

Your role, as an aide caring for a patient on an A.D.L. program, requires that you understand the following things:

> That good balance is needed to perform independent self-care.
> That any self-care activity is made up of many steps, and sometimes a patient must conquer these steps one by one.
> That the patient constantly needs your patience and encouragement.

You can best help your patient with A.D.L. activities by doing the following things:

Use the same words every day to instruct and encourage a patient. Make these words clear, simple, and brief.

Don't rush the patient. Allow him time to complete an activity at his own pace.

Find out if the patient is more interested in one activity than in another. Concentrate on the activity that interests him until he masters it.

See that the patient gets A.D.L. training at a time when he would normally perform that activity. (*Example:* If an incontinent patient usually has a bowel movement each morning after breakfast, bowel retraining should be done at that time.)

Allow the patient to do as much for himself as he is able.

Help him to master and use any adaptive equipment that may have been ordered for him.

See that adaptive equipment is in good working order and ready for the patient's use.

Position adaptive equipment so that the patient has easy access to it or can best use it.

A.D.L. Goals   *activities of Daily Living*

Goals for any patient on an A.D.L. program are individual and dependent on many factors other than those of the immediate physical problem.

Example: Two stroke patients have left-sided hemiplegia (paralysis of one side of the body).

One is a man of 68 who was an engineer and in good general health until the stroke occurred.
He has two sons and a daughter, living nearby, who visit, encourage, and help him.

The other, a woman, is 82. She had poor vision, a partial hearing loss, and an enlarged heart before the stroke occurred. She had worked in an insurance office before retirement at age 55. Her only relative is a niece who lives in another state and visits her once a year.

It is easy to see that the motivations and capabilities of these patients would be strong factors in the success of their A.D.L. retraining programs.

Something else that can influence the success of an A.D.L. program is the ability of the patient and staff to think of new ideas that suit the individual's needs.

Here are some of the many adaptive things that are used in A.D.L.

Moving about in bed
     rope pull (Fig. 15)
     trapeze
Personal grooming
     nail clipper
     suction cup nailbrush
     soap on a cord to wear around the neck
     bath mitt
     reachers to hold washcloth, powder puff, and other objects
     curlers of self-fastening material, such as Velcro
     long-handled bath brush or sponge
     bathtub seat with back rest
     wheelchair with commode seat for incontinent patient
     spray deodorant
     built-up handles on water faucets
Dressing and undressing
     long-handled clothing hook
     loops sewed on clothing for use with clothing hook
     larger sized clothing of stretch materials
     clothing with front openings
     trousers with elastic tops

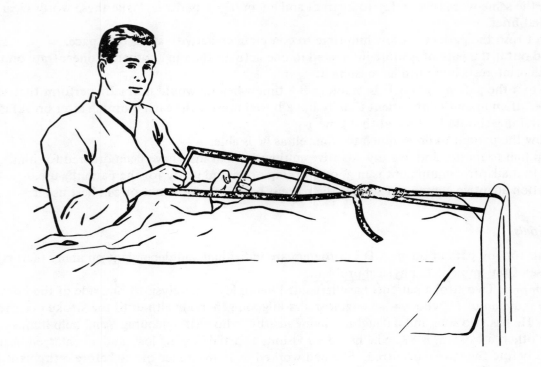

Figure 15. A self-help pulling device. (Reprinted by permission of © J. T. Posey Co.)

    Velcro self-closing fasteners
    large buttons
    a loop on the pull tab of a zipper
    device for putting on stockings (Fig. 16)
    elastic shoelaces
    long-handled shoe horn
    elastic cuff links

Eating
    utensils with built-up handles
    utensils with long handles
    utensils with rockers
    utensils with swivels
    A.D.L. palm cuff to hold various utensils
    drinking straws
    unbreakable dishes and glassware
    spillproof edges on dishes and glassware
    suction mat under dish to prevent slipping

Using the hands
    book rest
    page turner
    special telephone arms
    weighted pencils, checkers, and other objects

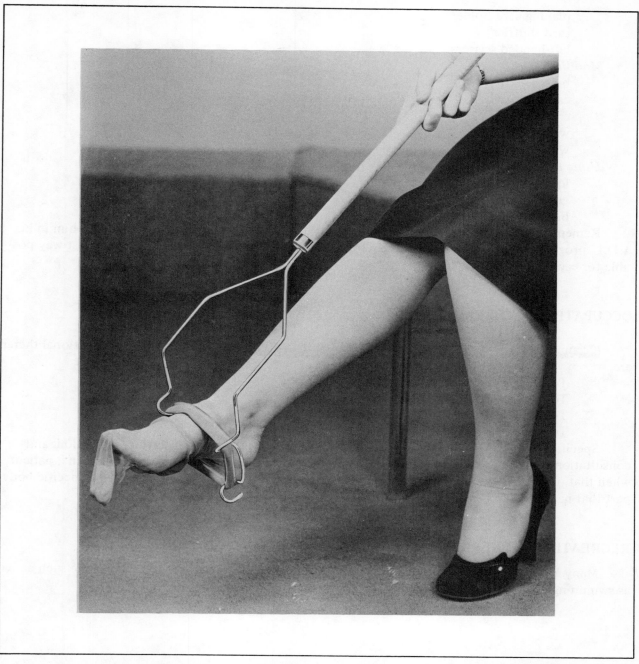

Figure 16. An A.D.L. self-care device. (Reprinted by permission of © J. A. Preston Corp., 1971.)

clip clothespin with peg (for holding pencil or pen)
embroidery hoop with table clamp
rubber doorknob lever
car door opener
easy-open coin purse
holder for knitting, crocheting, and other needlecrafts

playing card holder
card shuffler
left-handed scissors
Mobility
braces
canes
crutches
walkers
wheelchairs
Using the toilet
long-handled tongs for self-wiping
grab bars for toilet
built-up toilet seat

Remember that you have a great responsibility toward your patient in working with him in his A.D.L. program. The best and fastest way for you to work can only be the best and fastest way possible for each individual patient.

OCCUPATIONAL THERAPY

Occupational therapy is treatment by keeping the patient busy. The aims of occupational therapy are:

To occupy the mind and interest of a patient
To increase a patient's activity
To develop specific control of physical abilities
To train a patient for a job

Specific occupational therapy for the individual patient is given after testing, evaluation, and consultation with other staff members. Therapy such as tooling leather or weaving is given a patient when that occupation increases range of motion, strength, coordination, and agility in a specific body part that needs such rebuilding.

RECREATIONAL THERAPY

Many kinds of recreational therapy are also useful as physical therapy. These include such activities as swimming, bird-watching or nature walks, and games such as shuffle board.

6

YOUR GERIATRIC PATIENT NEEDS ADAPTIVE EQUIPMENT

STUDY GUIDE

What is adaptive equipment?

What two kinds of adaptive equipment are used?

Why should you become familiar with your patients' adaptive equipment?

What should you do if you notice a change in the condition of a piece of adaptive equipment or in the way a patient uses it?

What general rules should you follow when a patient has a piece of adaptive equipment?

Braces

What is a brace and why is it used?

What affects a patient's use of a brace?

If a patient wears a walking brace, what should be inspected along with the brace?

Why should the skin under a brace be examined and skin care given before and after the brace is worn?

What type of clothing should be worn with a brace?

What do you need in order to apply a brace?

Tell how to apply a short leg brace.

Canes

What should a geriatric patient have in order to use a cane?

For what two main purposes are canes used?

On which side is a cane carried, if it is used primarily for weight bearing?

How is a weight-bearing cane measured?

How is a weight-bearing cane used when walking?

On which side is a cane carried if it is used primarily for balance?

How is a balance cane measured?

How is it used in walking?

What two types of canes are common?

What should you do before a patient uses a cane?

What should you do while a patient is using a cane?

Corsets

Why is a corset ordered for a geriatric patient?

What are your general duties for a patient who wears a corset?

How do you help a patient put on a corset?

Crutches

Why would a doctor order a crutch for a patient?

What three types of crutches are common?

How do they differ?

Why is the axillary bar of a crutch always padded?

Why are rubber suction tips always used on crutch ends?

Why must the suction tips be cleaned regularly?

What six things should a crutch user do?

What is a gait pattern?

What are your responsibilities to the patient with a crutch?

Feeding Equipment

What is a feeding device?

Why is patience necessary when helping a patient with a feeding device?

What do you need when helping with feeding equipment?

Tell what you do when helping with feeding equipment.

Prostheses

What is a prosthesis?

Why is cleanliness of a prosthesis and the skin site so important?

What are your general duties to the patient with a prosthesis?

What general duties apply to the patient with an arm or leg prosthesis?

What do you need to help a patient put on a leg prosthesis?

What do you do to help the patient put on a leg prosthesis?

Walkers

What does the use of a walker accomplish?

Who orders the use of a walker?

What three types of walkers are common?

What do you do for a patient before he uses a walker?

What do you do while a patient is using a walker?

Wheelchairs

Who orders a wheelchair for a patient?

When should a patient not be allowed to use his wheelchair?

What types of wheelchairs are available?

What accessories are available for wheelchairs?

Tell how a wheelchair should be cleaned and maintained.

What are your general duties to the patient with a wheelchair?

ADAPTIVE EQUIPMENT

Adaptive equipment is any article that allows a patient to regain use of a body part or to perform a body function.

As a geriatric patient ages and becomes less and less able to function, he becomes more and more dependent on adaptive equipment to keep him active and caring for himself. For mobility he may require special shoes as his first equipment; then a walking cane and an eating device; then a leg brace; next a walker; then a standard wheelchair, a different eating device, and an arm brace; and last, a special wheelchair.

He nearly always needs glasses, and these are changed regularly to adapt to his failing vision.

Often, he may require a hearing aid.

Use of specific adaptive devices for care of special geriatric conditions may be found in the section The Healthier Body and Some Common Geriatric Conditions. (*Example:* Use of a hearing aid can be found in Caring for the Geriatric Patient with Loss of Hearing.)

Two main kinds of adaptive equipment are used:

   Standard — manufactured alike but selected for size or adjusted to the size of the individual.

   Custom — designed and made to suit the needs of the individual person.

While working as a geriatric aide, you will handle many pieces of both kinds of equipment. It is important for you to become familiar with every piece used by each of your patients. Then you can easily determine the following necessary information about adaptive equipment:

   If the equipment is working well or not.

   If the patient is using the equipment correctly or not.

   If the equipment no longer seems to suit the patient's needs.

Any change in the condition of a piece of equipment, a patient's technique of using it, or his ability to use it should be reported to the charge nurse as soon as it is observed.

Certain general rules apply to the use of any adaptive equipment or devices.

YOU DO THIS

Do not allow a patient to use a piece of equipment until he has been instructed in its safe and most effective use. This may be done by the nurse involved with activities of daily living (A.D.L.), the occupational therapist, the charge nurse, the physical therapist, or a combination of these people.

Know how to use a piece of equipment before helping a patient with its use.

Check every piece of equipment before and after use to determine its condition. If you cannot correct a defect, report it to the charge nurse.

Do not allow a patient to use a piece of defective equipment.

Check any complementary equipment to determine its condition. (*Example:* Check the patient's shoes if he uses a walker, and report a defect that you cannot correct.)

Keep a patient's personal equipment within his own room. See that is is marked with his name and room number.

Place equipment so that the patient has easy access to it.

Take care of a patient's personal needs, such as toileting, before equipment is used.

See that the patient is dressed to allow the best use of the equipment.

Position the patient in the best manner to use the equipment.

See that the patient uses the equipment as instructed.

Allow him ample time to use the equipment by himself.

Observe his use of equipment, and suggest changes for better use to the patient or charge nurse.

During use of equipment, check the patient's skin, where it contacts equipment, for indications of pulling or pinching from pressure.

Give special skin care before and after use of equipment to areas affected by use of equipment.

Report skin changes to the charge nurse.

Do not allow a patient to exhaust himself through use of equipment.

Clean equipment after use.

Besides equipment checks before and after use and cleaning after use, much adaptive equipment needs regular maintenance and repair. In nursing homes, this is usually done by specially trained mechanics.

BRACES

A brace is an adaptive appliance used to support the body or a body part (Fig. 17). The doctor is the one who always orders the use of a brace, and it is usually custom-made to fit a patient. A brace

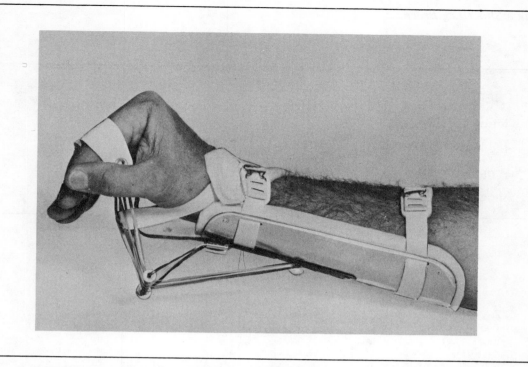

Figure 17. An arm brace. (Reprinted by permission of © J. A. Preston Corp., 1971.)

may be ordered to help a patient to walk, to control involuntary body movements, and to correct and prevent deformity. Careful handling of a brace is essential to maintain correct brace alignment. You should also remember that such an appliance is costly and that careful handling saves the patient unnecessary expense.

The individual patient's use of a brace is affected by:

      his desire to walk

      his attitude toward the brace

      the comfort of the brace

      whether the brace is correctly applied

A walking brace requires a special shoe to accommodate it, and both shoes and the brace should be inspected for signs of wear and need of repair before and after every wearing. It is best to leave the shoe attached to the brace.

The skin must be examined frequently for pressure areas caused by contact with a brace, and skin care given before and after each use of the brace. Signs of pressure should be reported to the charge nurse immediately.

Clothing to be worn over a brace must be large and loose enough to accommodate the brace without strain. If the patient removes the brace during the day, it may be best for him to wear the brace outside of his clothing.

Encourage the patient to do as much as he can toward applying the brace by himself. Allow him ample time.

YOU NEED
>   lotion for skin care
>
>   the brace (Fig. 18)
>
>   supportive shoes
>
>   shoehorn

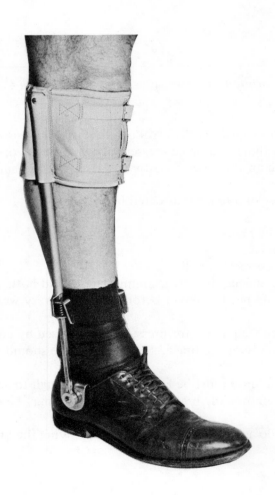

Figure 18.   A leg brace. (Reprinted by permission of © J. A. Preston Corp., 1971.)

YOU DO THIS

Position the patient lying or sitting in bed with legs extended.

Give skin care to areas that contact the brace. Check skin for signs of pressure.

Put on sock or stocking that is free of holes or mends and that fits the foot without wrinkling.

Attach shoe to brace, if necessary.

Tuck brace straps out of the way.

Slightly bend patient's knee. Place brace under lower part of leg, guiding foot into shoe and making sure that patient's toes do not curl under.

Use shoehorn, if necessary, to see that heel is securely in shoe.

Lace shoe and tie securely.

Fasten straps, allowing enough space to insert two fingers beneath brace fastenings. If the brace has an ankle strap, fasten it around the outside of the opposite upright (strip of metal).

Check leg for signs of pressure by brace.

Put other shoe on patient before helping him off the bed.

CANES

A cane is often the first walking aid used by a geriatric patient. Good control of the body trunk and strength in the arm and hand are necessary for a patient to use one. A cane is ordered by the doctor to suit the need of the patient and is measured to suit that need. A patient needs a cane that serves one of two main purposes. They are:

    primarily to bear weight
    primarily to maintain balance

If a cane is used primarily for weight bearing, it is carried on the same side as the weak leg. A cane for this purpose is measured so that the patient's arm is stiff when bearing weight on the cane. When the patient walks, the cane is advanced, a step is made with the good leg, and weight is borne by the cane while the weak leg is brought forward.

If a cane is used primarily for balance, the cane is carried on the side opposite the weak leg. This cane is measured to allow for a 30-degree bend of the elbow. When the patient walks, the cane is moved forward before a step is made with the weak leg.

Two types of canes are common.

    Standard – a bent-handled cane available in several kinds of wood and aluminum.

    Four-legged – an aluminum cane with a shovel type of handgrip and four legs (Fig. 19).

Regardless of the type of cane used and the main purpose, you have specific responsibilities to the patient.

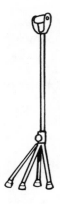

Figure 19. A four-legged cane. (From Elementary Rehabilitation Nursing Care, *U.S. Public Health Service, Division of Nursing.)*

YOU DO THIS

Before Use

    Check patient's shoes for signs of wear or need of repair.

    Be sure shoes fit well and are tied securely.

    Check the cane tips and replace worn rubber suction tips. Clean tips if necessary.

    Check the cane for loose screws, cracks, or splinters.

    Report any defects to the charge nurse.

During Use

    See that the patient stands as straight as possible and looks straight ahead, not at his feet.

    See that he carries the cane on the side for which it is ordered.

A Loftstrand or Canadian crutch is often used as a substitute for a cane (Fig. 20). Your duties concerning its use are the same as for a cane. (*See* Crutches.)

CORSETS

A corset may be ordered for a geriatric patient to help support his back and trunk and to give better balance.

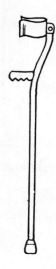

Figure 20. Loftstrand or Canadian crutch. (From Elementary Rehabilitation Nursing Care, *U.S. Public Health Service, Division of Nursing.)*

Your General Duties to a Patient with a Corset

YOU DO THIS

Give special skin care before and after use. Report signs of irritation or pressure to the charge nurse.

Inspect corset for broken, bent, or worn spots. Report any defect to the charge nurse.

See that the corset is clean and dry.

See that a patient's bony areas are padded to prevent irritation from corset stays.

See that undergarments are worn over the corset to allow for easier use of the toilet.

Helping a Patient Put on a Corset

YOU NEED

corset

padding material, if necessary. (Self-adhering foam is good.)

Help the patient to lay on his side.

Underroll the far side of the corset halfway.

Place the roll against the patient's spine so that the middle two stays of the back of the corset support the spine. Position the corset low under the buttocks because it tends to ride up when the patient sits.

Tuck the rolled half of the corset under the patient's body.

Hold the corset in place while turning the patient onto his back.

Bring the ends of the corset together in front.

See that the sides are even and that the lower edge of the corset is placed just over the pubic bone.

Smooth the lower edge under the buttocks.

Fasten the corset, working upward from the lower edge and smoothing wrinkles from under the flaps.

Check the corset for correct space by inserting two fingers in the top of the corset when the patient is in a sitting position. If the corset is too tight or too loose, report it to the charge nurse.

CRUTCHES

A crutch or crutches may be ordered by the doctor for a patient after amputation, fracture, operation, or injury to a leg.

Three types are common.

Loftstrand or Canadian. Usually custom-made, it fits the forearm by means of a metal cuff and is made of aluminum.

A patient is measured for a Loftstrand crutch, by adjusting the cuff and handgrip, so that his elbow is bent at about a 30-degree angle and the crutch tip extends 6–8 inches to the side of his foot.

Loftstrand crutches are preferred because they allow a patient to adjust his clothes or to take hold of another object without losing the use of the crutch. They also eliminate the pressure on ribs and armpits that is unavoidable with the axillary crutch. They are often used instead of canes.

Standard axillary. Nonadjustable, it fits into the patient's armpit and is usually made of wood.

Extension axillary. Adjustable, it fits into the patient's armpit and may be made of wood or aluminum (Fig. 21).

A patient is fitted for axillary crutches by measuring the length from the patient's armpit to a point 6 inches out from the side of the sole of his foot, or by measuring the length from the patient's armpit to the side of the sole of his foot and adding 2 inches. Handgrips are adjusted so that the patient's elbows are bent at about 30-degree angles.

The axillary bar of a crutch is always padded to prevent undue pressure on ribs and armpits.

MEETING YOUR GERIATRIC PATIENT'S NEEDS

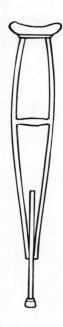

Figure 21. Extension axillary adjustable crutch. (From Elementary Rehabilitation Nursing Care, *U.S. Public Health Service, Division of Nursing.)*

All crutches have rubber suction tips that prevent slipping. These are replaceable and must be checked regularly for signs of wear. Tips sometimes collect dirt and dust that cause them to slip. They must be cleaned regularly. When using a crutch, a patient should do the following:

Stand as straight as possible.

Look straight ahead, not at his feet.

Hug the axillary bar close to the body against the rib cage.

Maintain enough space between armpit and top of crutch to insert two horizontally held fingers.

Bear body weight on hands, never on armpits, to prevent possible paralysis of hand and arm.

To allow for the correct three points of support base, never have the crutches and feet in the same line.

A patient is instructed in the safe and correct use of crutches. He is taught one or more of the following gait patterns:

Four point. Move right crutch, left foot; left crutch, right foot. It is a simple, slow, but safe method; there are always three points of support on the floor.

Two point. Move right crutch and left foot simultaneously, then left crutch and right foot simultaneously. This requires more balance than the four-point method because only two points are supporting the body at any one time.

Three point. Move both crutches and the weaker lower extremity forward simultaneously and then move the stronger lower extremity forward. It is used when one lower extremity cannot take full or any weight bearing and the other extremity can support the whole body weight.

Tripod alternate. Move right crutch, left crutch; drag feet forward. This method is used by those unable to lift either extremity.

Tripod simultaneous (rocking horse gait). Move both crutches forward simultaneously; drag feet forward. This method is also used by those unable to lift either extremity.

Swinging to. Move both crutches forward; then lift and swing body forward just short of the crutches.

Swinging through. Move both crutches forward; then lift and swing body beyond crutches. Skill, strength, and proper timing are required. Use swinging gait to lift body off the floor when there is a severe disability of the lower extremities.

Sideward four point. Move right crutch to right; right foot to right; left foot to right; left crutch to right.

Backward four point. Move left foot back; right crutch back; right foot back; left crutch back.

Turning on crutches. Place one crutch in front of body, the other slightly to the side and rear; pivot feet or lift body in direction crutches were moved. Repeat as often as necessary to make turn.

Your Responsibilities to the Patient with a Crutch

YOU DO THIS

Before Use

Check patient's shoes for signs of wear or need of repair.

Be sure shoes fit well and are tied securely.

Check crutch tips and replace worn rubber suction tips. Clean tips if necessary.

Check crutch for axillary padding, loose screws, cracks, or splinters.

Report a defect to the charge nurse.

During Use

See that the patient stands straight and looks ahead, not at his feet (Fig. 22)

See that he uses the crutch as taught.

After Use

Check the body areas that contact the crutch for signs of pressure. Give special skin care to these areas.

FEEDING EQUIPMENT OR DEVICES

A feeding device is an appliance that is fitted to a hand or arm that has lost some function and allows the patient to feed himself with little or no assistance. A patient with limited range of motion or muscle weakness might require such a device.

Patience is of the utmost importance when helping a patient with special feeding equipment. It may take him a long time to complete a meal, especially when he is just learning to use the device. Encourage him and allow him plenty of time to use the equipment by himself, but do not let him become exhausted by his attempts or go hungry. Feed him if necessary.

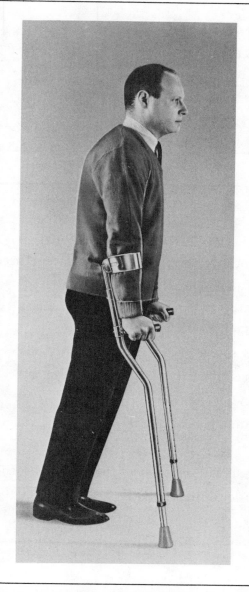

Figure 22.   A patient correctly using Loftstrand crutches. (Reprinted by permission of © J. A. Preston Corp., 1971.)

Helping with Feeding Equipment

YOU NEED

the patient's feeding device

special silverware

plate guard

suction under mat for holding plate

rocker arm, overhead sling, or balancer

special straws

bib or napkin

YOU DO THIS

See that the patient is in a comfortable sitting position.

Place his arm in the rocker, overhead sling, or balancer if needed.

Put his bib or napkin around his neck.

Attach the feeding device and allow the patient a few practice swings with it to be sure he can reach both the plate and his mouth.

Position the food tray so that the patient has the best access to it.

Prepare food, such as cutting meat or buttering bread, as necessary.

Put the food guard on the plate.

Be sure liquids are within patient's reach.

Put straws in liquids.

Allow the patient to eat with as much independence as possible.

Allow the patient sufficient time to eat.

Help him if necessary.

PROSTHESES

A prosthesis is a device fitted to the body to replace a part that is missing. Artificial limbs, artificial eyes, and dentures are examples of external prostheses. Artificial femur heads, artificial blood vessels or heart valves, and cardiac pacemakers are examples of surgically implanted internal prostheses.

Cleanliness and daily care of a prosthesis and the amputation or extraction site are of utmost importance. Skin and membranes are easily irritated by contact with prostheses, and when an inflammation or rash occurs, use of a prosthesis may be suspended by the doctor.

Your General Duties to the Patient with a Prosthesis

YOU DO THIS

Report to the charge nurse if the patient complains of pain, pressure, or pinching from a prosthesis.

Check the prosthetic area before and after use for redness, rash, bruises, or swelling.

Check the prosthesis before and after use for loose, worn, bent, broken, or stiff parts.

Report a defect of the prosthetic side of the patient or the prosthesis to the charge nurse at once.

If the Prosthesis Is a Leg or an Arm

Give special skin care before and after use of prosthesis.

See that the patient has a supply of stump socks.

See that he wears a stump sock when using the prosthesis and afterward, except for airing periods. (Stump socks help to prevent swelling.)

Be sure that the stump sock is kept smooth and wrinkle-free to prevent creasing of the skin.

See that the patient is dressed in clothes that allow easy use of the prosthesis. Trousers should be reinforced at the side where they contact a knee bolt and sleeves at the side where they rub against an elbow bolt. A cotton stocking should be worn under a nylon stocking to prevent runs due to the prosthesis.

Check stump socks for worn spots. Report such spots to the charge nurse. These indicate a need for correction of the prosthesis by a specialist.

Helping a Patient Put on a Leg Prosthesis

YOU NEED

stump sock

prosthesis

strong straight chair

YOU DO THIS

Help the patient to a standing position, facing you.

Allow him to support himself by holding onto the back of a straight chair. (The side of amputation should be closest to the chair.)

See that the stump sock is clean, dry, and smooth. Draw it well up on the stump.

Place the prosthesis under the stump so that the toe is positioned outward.

Steady the prosthesis foot against the leg of the chair.

Push the stump into the socket.

Fasten the pelvic belt. (This turns the toe of the prosthesis inward to a normal position.)

Be sure the pelvic belt is horizontal and cannot ride up over the hip of the normal leg.

Smooth the sock at the top of the prosthesis.

WALKERS

A walker offers a secure cage within which a patient can move without fear of falling. No patient should be allowed to use a walker unless a doctor has ordered its use. The walker is adjusted to the size and needs of the patient and he is instructed in its safe use. Elbows should be bent at 30-degree angles when the patient uses the walker.

Three types of walkers are common.

Standard — a rigid four-legged frame used as an aid for balance and weight bearing when walking. It requires use of safety suction tips. The patient's weight is thrown alternately to the front and back of the walker as he steps (Fig. 23).

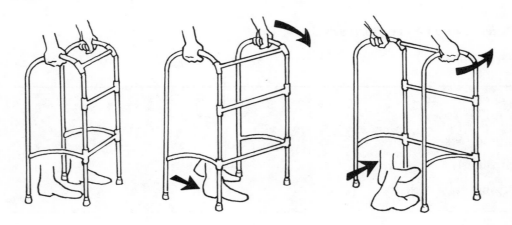

Figure 23. Proper use of a walker. (From Elementary Rehabilitation Nursing Care, *U.S. Public Health Service, Division of Nursing.)*

MEETING YOUR GERIATRIC PATIENT'S NEEDS

Gliding — a standard frame, adapted by putting button casters on the walker's metal tips. The patient is able to push the walker and still maintain good control. (Wheels on walkers have proved to be unsafe.)

Reciprocal — a hinged frame that allows the patient to move it forward one side at a time. It requires use of safety suction tips.

Your General Duties to the Patient Who Uses a Walker

YOU DO THIS

Before Use

Check patient's shoes for signs of wear or need of repair.

Be sure shoes are on correctly and are tied securely.

Check walker tips and replace worn rubber tips if needed. Clean tips if necessary.

Check walker for loose screws or defective parts.

Report a defect to the charge nurse immediately.

During Use

See that the patient stands as straight as possible and looks ahead, not at his feet.

See that he uses the walker as taught. The patient is often fearful and needs reminding to maintain correct weight bearing and feet positionings.

WHEELCHAIRS

Wheelchairs are ordered by the doctor for patients with a variety of handicaps, and many factors are considered in selecting the proper chair and accessories for the individual. The techniques of using a wheelchair also vary according to the individual patient's needs. The patient should not be allowed to use his wheelchair until he has been instructed in its use.

Types of Wheelchairs

Universal. This chair has larger wheels in the back. It can be used indoors and outdoors; it ensures better posture, allows easier transfer activities, and can be tilted to go up curbs and stairs.

Traveler. This chair has larger wheels in front. It is used only indoors and on level surfaces; it allows poorer posture, is more difficult for transferring activities, and cannot be used for curbs or stairs.

Amputee. This chair has the rear wheels set back. It maintains safe balance by compensating for loss of the patient's weight in front due to amputation. Footrests and legrests are available for a one-sided amputee or a patient wearing a prosthesis.

One-arm drive. This chair has both handrims on one side. It may be prescribed for those who have only one good arm, such as the hemiplegic or the amputee. This chair is too wide for most doors, and it is difficult to learn to use.

Power-driven. This chair is propelled by a motor. It should be used only by patients with no possible means of propelling themselves.

Custom. This chair is designed for a specific patient.

Geriatric patients sometimes use two other kinds of wheelchairs. One is a small, strong, straight chair with caster wheels on the leg tips. This can be ordered in metal or adapted from a wooden kitchen chair. The other type is a commode wheelchair with an open seat and a removable waste pan for use by incontinent patients.

Sizes of Wheelchairs

Wheelchairs are made in four sizes:
    adult
    adult, extra wide
    junior
    child

Accessories

A patient's disabilities and potential abilities determine which accessories are ordered for his wheelchair.

Brakes. Every wheelchair should be equipped with brakes for the safety of the patient.

Wheels. Front casters that are 5 inches in diameter are standard equipment on wheelchairs; however, the 8-inch caster allows for better patient control of the wheelchair. Handrims with multiple grasp projections may be used by a patient who is unable to hold a regular handrim.

Armrests. Upholstered armrests allow greater comfort. Removable arms may be needed so that the patient can transfer in and out of the chair. Armrests may be equipped with button brake locks. Desk arms may be ordered if accessibility to a desk or table is necessary.

Backrests. Adjustable backrests may be ordered for the patient who is unable to sit in an upright position all the time. Zippered backrests may be ordered for a patient who must be transferred to and from the chair by being slid in and out of the back. Removable headrests may be ordered for additional back and head support.

Legrests. Adjustable legrests may be ordered for the patient who must have one or both legs elevated. Swinging detachable legrests may be ordered to allow the patient a closer approach in transferring.

Footrests. Heel loops, which prevent the feet from slipping off the footrest, may be ordered for one or both feet. A two-heel strap may be used if both feet must be held on the footrest. Toe loops for maintaining foot position may be ordered.

Seat cushions. Foam rubber seat cushions 2—4 inches thick are used for the patient's comfort and for prevention of pressure sores.

Care of Wheelchairs

Proper care of a wheelchair is important. Regular attention keeps a wheelchair in good condition and prolongs its usefulness.

Cleaning. Wipe all metal parts of the wheelchair once a week with a light coating of general purpose household oil applied with a soft cloth. Wipe leather or plastic upholstery with a damp cloth and clean with saddle soap. Be sure to dry both chrome and leather whenever they are wet.

Lubrication. Oil the center bolt of the crossbars and the point of attachment of the brakes to the lower side bars. Grease both front and rear wheel axles with petroleum jelly or any grease lubricant.

(This is generally necessary only once a year.) Apply paraffin wax when needed to any telescoping parts, such as adjustable backs, removable arms, footrests, and extensions. DO NOT OIL OR GREASE THESE PARTS.

Miscellaneous. Be sure to keep nuts, bolts, screws, and other fastening devices tight, and if any part breaks, have it repaired by an authorized wheelchair repairman. Be sure to use a wheelchair wrench for adjusting footrests.

Using a Wheelchair

A patient can manipulate a standard wheelchair by using both arms or by using one arm and one leg.

Using Both Arms

Moving forward. Grasp the handrims as far toward the back of the wheels as possible and push both wheels forward at the same time. Long, even pushes are less tiring than short, erratic ones.

Turning. To turn a corner, push the wheel on the opposite side from the direction you want to turn and hold the other wheel still. To turn around in a small space, place one hand forward on one handrim and the other hand back on the opposite handrim; pull with the forward hand and at the same time push with the back hand.

Using One Arm and One Leg

Moving forward. Pushing only one wheel turns the chair in a circle; therefore, push the wheel with the good hand and at the same time use the good foot to oppose and counter the turn and allow the chair to go forward.

Turning. To turn toward the affected side, use only the opposite hand to turn the wheelchair. To turn toward the unaffected side, reach across to the opposite wheel with the good hand and, use the good foot in the same way as in the forward movement.

Your General Duties to the Patient with a Wheelchair

YOU DO THIS

Keep the chair and pillow supports clean.

Inspect the chair before and after use for loose or improperly working parts.

Report any defect to the head nurse immediately.

Help the patient in transferring to and from the wheelchair.

See that the patient is positioned correctly in the chair and maintains good sitting alignment.

See that the safety belt is fastened.

If the patient is in the chair for long periods, see that he changes position or exercises from time to time.

See that brake locks are on whenever the chair is not moving.

Release the brake to wheel the chair.

When you wheel a chair, be sure the patient's elbows are inside the armrests.

When you wheel a chair through a doorway, turn the chair around so that you go first and pull the chair after you.

When you wheel a chair to descend from a curb, turn the chair around and lower the back wheels off the curb first.

When you park a patient in a wheelchair, be sure the chair is in a place where it will not interfere with traffic.

Never park a patient so that he faces a wall or can be troubled by unseen activity behind him.

MEETING YOUR GERIATRIC PATIENT'S NEEDS

7

YOUR GERIATRIC PATIENT NEEDS REMOTIVATION AND RESOCIALIZATION

STUDY GUIDE

What is remotivation?

What is resocialization?

When are remotivation and resocialization necessary?

How does aging affect a geriatric patient's motivation and socialization?

What can happen to the aged person who is not remotivated or resocialized?

Whose duty is it to remotivate and resocialize a geriatric patient?

What two departments of a nursing facility do most of the work of remotivation and resocialization?

What does an occupational therapist do?

What does a recreational therapist do?

What are the duties of all nursing personnel toward occupational and recreational therapies?

What are your duties as geriatric aide toward a patient in an occupational and recreational program?

What special remotivation and resocialization techniques should you and all geriatric nursing personnel use?

What should you do when speaking to any patient?

What should you do when any patient speaks to you?

What should you do when any patient joins a group?

How can you orient a patient to the day of the week?

How can you orient a patient to the time of the year?

How can you orient a patient to his location?

How can you keep a patient in touch with daily happenings inside and outside the nursing facility?

How can you help a patient take pride in himself?

How can you encourage a patient to talk to you?

How should you offer a choice to a patient?

With whom should you try to put your patient when he is joining a group?

Tell how you might conduct a resocialization and remotivation class for a small group of confused patients.

How long should such a class last?

How should such a class end?

REMOTIVATION is the process of renewing a person's urge to live and stimulating his desire to be active and to learn.

RESOCIALIZATION is the process of renewing a person's awareness of others and stimulating his desire and ability to participate in groups.

Both remotivation and resocialization are necessary on a daily, hour-to-hour basis throughout the lifetime of every person, from the loving encouragement of a baby's first steps, to the rewarded successes of adult life. The geriatric patient, though still in need of frequent encouragement, usually receives less and less.

Aging reduces the contact between a geriatric patient and the world. Communication problems, such as faulty vision, failing hearing and brain damage, make social relationships difficult. Lessening ability to move about, disease, and lowered income restrict an older person's activities. Deaths of family members and long-time friends deprive him of those who knew him best and shared his life and interests.

Because of these things and because the aging mind tends to forget present events and to recall the past, a patient often withdraws into himself, becomes lonely, depressed, and loses interest in life. If allowed to continue in this state of mind, he deteriorates into total dependency and untimely death.

It is important then that a geriatric patient be stimulated into activities and social relationships. Such stimulation is called remotivation and resocialization. It is one of the main duties of all personnel in a geriatric nursing facility.

OCCUPATIONAL AND RECREATIONAL THERAPIES

Much of the work of remotivation and resocialization is done by two departments within a nursing facility. They are the departments of occupational and recreational therapy.

An occupational therapist trains a patient and provides him with work and creative activities designed for his particular abilities and talents. Through occupational therapy he gains self-satisfaction and the esteem of others. He feels capable, functioning, necessary, and admired.

Despite handicaps, his abilities may allow him to perform several complicated jobs. He may do part-time typing in the office of the nursing facility, where he works among full-time nonresident employees. The patient may do doll repairing and dressing in the occupational therapy room, where he works with other patients, and he may make an afghan in the privacy of his room. Or he may be limited to a bedside job that would be easy for a child but is difficult for him, with only the visits of the occupational therapist and the nursing staff to sustain and encourage him. (*See* Your Geriatric Patient Needs Physical Therapy.)

The word *recreate* means *to begin anew.* That is the design and intention of recreational therapy. The recreational therapist plans social events, distractions, and pleasures that refresh and renew the patient's mind, body, and emotions (Fig. 24.) Some of these may be quiet, solitary pleasures, such as reading; others may be physically active and competitive, such as shuffleboard. Still others may be parties, lectures, and theater trips that enrich the social and mental life of the patient.

Because of the importance of occupational and recreational therapies, all nursing personnel have the responsibility to see that each patient participates in these programs, that whenever possible a

Activities

87th STREET RESIDENCE

FOR THE WEEK OF JUNE 14 - JUNE 18

MONDAY, JUNE 14

| 10:00-12:00 A.M. | ARTS AND CRAFTS
MISS HILLINGER WILL NOT BE HERE TODAY | 2ND FLOOR |
| 3:00 P.M. | READING CIRCLE | 4TH FLOOR |

TUESDAY, JUNE 15

11:00 A.M.	CURRENT EVENTS	4TH FLOOR
2:00 P.M.	CARD GAMES - FOR MEN	2ND FLOOR
2:45 P.M.	FUN MUSIC HOUR - WITH SYLVIA RESNICK	4TH FLOOR
6:30 P.M.	MOVIE	FRONT DINING- ROOM

WEDNESDAY, JUNE 16

| 10:00-12:00 A.M. | ARTS AND CRAFTS
WITH MISS HILLINGER | 2ND FLOOR |
| 12:00 noon | BAR-B-Q | GARDEN AT
87TH STREET |

THURSDAY, JUNE 17

10:00-12-00 A.M.	ARTS AND CRAFTS	2ND FLOOR
3:00 P.M.	BINGO	FRONT DINING- ROOM
7:30 P.M.	VALLY WEIGL - MUSIC PROGRAM	4TH FLOOR

FRIDAY, JUNE 18

| 1:30-5:00 P.M. | ARTS AND CRAFTS
WITH MISS HILLINGER | 2ND FLOOR |
| 6:45 P.M. | SABBATH SERVICES | 4TH FLOOR |

Figure 24.   Sample recreational activities sheet.

patient's nursing care plan does not conflict with these programs, and that the patient's interests and efforts in every program are encouraged.

As an aide, you must see that your patients are aware of and attend scheduled programs. You must talk with them about what they are doing. You must praise them for good work or improvement, and you must help them if necessary.

SPECIAL TECHNIQUES

You and all nursing personnel have other more important remotivational and resocializational duties than just cooperation with occupational and recreational therapies. It is your duty to maintain and stimulate contact with the minds of your patients. In your numerous daily contacts with your patients you must use special techniques that orient a patient to the present, future and past, to his location, to who he is, to whom he is with, and to what is expected of him. In other sections of this book specific examples are given for use under certain conditions.

Here are some general rules.

When speaking to a patient:

Speak slowly and distinctly.

Use a normal, clear voice. Don't shout.

Use direct, short sentences.

Look directly into the patient's face and give him your complete attention. Smile.

Take hold of the patient's hand or otherwise touch him.

Always mention his name.

Always mention your name.

Be friendly. Never scold him.

Repeat your statements as often as necessary.

When a patient speaks to you:

Listen.

Don't rush him.

Don't ignore him or pass by him.

Never laugh at him.

If you don't understand him, ask him simple questions to determine what he wants.

When a patient is joining a group:

Tell him where he is going and what will happen there.

Example: "Mrs. Smith, it's Mrs. Caldwell. Shall we go to the dining room for lunch?"

Mention the names of all members of the group, including the patient.

Example: "Hi there, Mr. Brown, Mrs. Jones, Miss Jackson. Here is Mr. Smith to join you. Have a nice lunch everybody."

Whenever possible, mention the general time of day.

Examples: "Good morning" or "Lunch time;"

"Your favorite nighttime television program will be on in a few minutes."

Whenever possible, mention the day of the week.

Example: "It's Friday. Your favorite nighttime television program will be on in a few minutes."

Whenever possible, mention the season or month.

Example: "It's nice to have television on a cold January night."

Whenever possible, mention the place where the patient is.

Examples: You have one of the nicest rooms at Cadbury House."

"Isn't it nice here on the sun porch?"

Whenever possible, mention events occurring within the facility.

Examples: "Did you enjoy the birthday party?"

"Are you going to the lecture?"

Whenever possible, mention current events.

Examples: "President Nixon is going to be on television."

"Aren't you from Connecticut? Your state has been in the news lately."

Whenever possible, compliment the patient on something he is doing or wearing.

Examples: "You certainly have learned how to manage your wheelchair."

"That shade of blue in your dress is so pretty with your blue eyes."

Whenever possible, get the patient to make a comment.

Example: "What do you think about it?"

When offering a choice to a patient, make the choice clear.

Example: Don't say "What would you like to do?"

Do say, "Would you like to go out on the sun porch, or would you like to go to the television room?"

STIMULATE CONVERSATION AMONG PATIENTS

Try to put a patient into a group that is on an equal or a slightly higher mental level. Try not to put him with a group in which most of the others are on a lower mental level.

Many nursing facilities offer classes in remotivation and resocialization for small groups of confused patients. Aides often conduct or participate in the programs, which are geared to levels of understanding.

On the lowest level a class may be conducted like this:

A group of six confused patients are brought to a nondistracting room and placed in comfortable chairs around a table on which are simple cooking components such as a pot, an egg beater, an apron, and an egg. At least four of the group should be more alert than the other two.

The person conducting the class stands by the table and smiles a greeting to each arrival. When all are assembled, the lecturer greets them and tells his name, repeating it frequently.

Example: "Good afternoon, ladies. It was so nice of you to come to the cooking class this afternoon. You know me, I'm Mrs. Smith. Mrs. Smith who teaches the cooking class."

The lecturer goes to each two patients in turn, shakes hands, calls the patients by name, and introduces them to each other.

Example: "Good afternoon, Mrs. Jones. Good afternoon Mrs. Jackson. Do you know each other? Mrs. Jones, this is Mrs. Jackson. Mrs. Jackson, this is Mrs. Jones."

When all have been introduced, the lecturer goes to the table, picks up the apron, holds it so all can see it, and asks, "Who can tell me what this is?" The lecturer allows plenty of time for answers, responds to those that come spontaneously, and speaks specifically and by name to those who don't reply.

Example: Mrs. Jones, when you cooked, did you use this?"

When response has been evoked, the lecturer puts on the apron and picks up the next item until all items have been seen, have evoked comment, and their use demonstrated: A good class could climax in a discussion by all of favorite foods and even of recipes.

After the class, which, to prevent fatigue, should last only 20 minutes, refreshments should be served. These should be definite treat or reward foods, not just the usual midmorning or midafternoon nourishment. Ice cream, pudding, a special cake, and special fruit are suitable.

Through the use of such remotivational and resocializational classes, many patients have returned to social awareness after years of confusion, isolation, and loneliness. Through references to past experiences and achievements, patients are able to establish contact with and function in the present, and even to look forward to the future.

In classes on a higher mental level, patients often have responsibility for the program, collect the necessary props, and take turns in conducting classes on familiar subjects about which each has special knowledge. (*Examples:* a trip to Washington or growing pansies.) They may even make and serve the refreshments.

Always remember that no patient is only an object for which you must take care, but a human being with whom you must make contact.

Create a climate of acceptance. This means making each patient in a group feel welcome and secure with you and with each other.

Create a bridge to reality. This means talking with them about generally familiar things.

Share the world we live in. This means drawing patients into conversation. Get them to comment on the general topic you have introduced.

Get them to appreciate the work of the world. This means stimulating patients to desire to work with you and each other.

Create a climate of appreciation. This means responding to and enjoying what patients contribute. Get them to elaborate on comments of their own and others.

8

YOUR GERIATRIC PATIENT NEEDS OBSERVATION AND TREATMENTS

STUDY GUIDE

On what does a definition of normal health always depend?

On what is a definition of health in a geriatric patient based?

Does all a person's body age at the same rate?

Why is it important to notice signs of aging?

How does aging affect resistance to illness?

What three things should help you to observe a geriatric patient?

How does aging affect a body in recognizable ways?

Symptoms

What are symptoms?

What are symptoms called when they are confined to a small body area?

What are symptoms called when they indicate that the entire body is affected?

Why is it important to report the date and the hour together with any symptoms?

Why is it important to report the exact location and description of any symptom?

Tell the correct way to report about a pain in a patient's leg.

Who should interpret symptoms?

How would you report symptoms that might suggest a cold?

Name some things about a patient to watch for and describe.

Name some things about a patient to listen for and describe.

Name some things about a patient to touch and describe.

Name some things that you can get your patient to tell you.

Vital Signs

What are vital signs?

What does taking body temperature help to do?

How often should temperature be taken?

How are body temperature, pulse, and respiration counts (TPRs) recorded?

Name three ways to take body temperature.

Tell how to take an oral temperature.

What is the normal oral temperature?

How long should a thermometer remain in the mouth?

Tell how to take a rectal temperature.

When should a rectal temperature be taken?

What is the normal rectal temperature?

How long should a thermometer remain in the rectum?

What kind of thermometer can be used to take an axillary temperature?

Tell how to take an axillary temperature.

How long should an axillary thermometer be left in place?

What is the normal axillary temperature?

Tell four important things to remember about glass thermometers.

What would you do if a glass thermometer were to break in a patient's mouth?

How frequently should the temperature of a geriatric patient be taken?

What materials do you need in order to take a temperature?

Tell step by step how you would take the temperature of a patient with a glass thermometer.

Tell how an electric skin thermometer is used.

Tell how a disposable oral thermometer is used.

Tell how to count the pulse.

Tell how to count respirations.

Where are TPRs recorded?

In what color is temperature usually charted? Pulse count?

Blood Pressure

Tell how to take a blood pressure reading.

Tubes, Tubing, and Other Equipment Used in Treatments

How are tubes used?

What tubes may be inserted by aides?

What is a rectal tube and how is it used? An enema tube? A douche nozzle?

What three general rules should you follow when using these tubes?

What four general rules should you follow when watching tubes or tubing?

How can a blocked tube be cleared of blockage?

How can you tell if a tube is disposable or not?

How do you clean and sterilize nondisposable tubes?

Applying Heat and Cold

How can heat and cold treatments be given?

What does a heat treatment do?

In what three ways can external heat be given?

How is dry heat given? Moist heat? Medicinal heat?

How does cold affect the body?

In what three ways can external cold be applied?

Why can application of heat or cold be dangerous to the geriatric patient?

What general rules should you follow when applying heat or cold to a geriatric patient.

How hot should the water be that is used to fill a hot water bottle for a geriatric patient?

Tell how to fill a hot water bottle.

Why should you always put a cover on a hot water bottle?

How do you care for a hot water bottle when it is not in use?

What is a hydrocollator steam pack?

Tell what you need to apply a hydrocollator steam pack?

Tell how to apply a hydrocollator steam pack.

Tell how to fill an ice bag. How full should it be?

How do you care for an ice bag when it is not in use?

Changing a Dressing

Who should change sterile dressings?

What do you need in order to change dressings?

Tell how to change dressings.

Why should you wear disposable gloves when changing dressings?

Why should dressings be put into a disposable bag?

What should you report for charting?

Applying an Elastic Bandage or Stocking

When is an elastic bandage used?

How can you determine what size bandage to use?

How should the bandage be applied?

What should you watch for in a patient wearing an elastic bandage?

What should you do if swelling occurs or if the skin becomes blue and cold?

How often should the bandage be removed and what care should be given the skin when the bandage is off?

Tell how to wash an elastic bandage or elastic stocking.

Tell how to apply an elastic bandage to an ankle.

Tell how to put on an elastic or support stocking.

Putting on an Arm Sling

Tell how to apply an arm sling.

Why should the knot at the back of the neck be to one side of the spine?

Why should the fingers of the arm in the sling be exposed?

Applying Binders and Restraints

For what purposes are binders used?

Who should order a binder or restraint?

What five things should you remember when putting on a binder?

Tell how to put a scultetus binder on a patient.

Tell how to put on a T-strap binder.

When are restraints used on a patient?

What parts of the body should be restrained to prevent a patient from getting out of bed?

What should you do before applying restraints?

What should you watch for after restraints have been applied?

How often should restraints be removed?

What sort of skin care should you give during the time the restraints are temporarily removed?

Tell how to use a length of material as a restraint.

How tight should the restraint knot be around the wrist or ankle?

Why should gauze or ropes never be used for restraints?

Tell how to make a restraint knot. A square knot.

When are mitt restraints used?

OBSERVING THE GERIATRIC PATIENT

Although the techniques for observing and recording symptoms are the same for any patient, regardless of age, a definition of normal health always depends on age. What is normal for a two-year-old is not normal for an adult. What is normal for an adult is not normal for an old person.

The normal, expected body behavior of an old person is one of gradual breakdown and decreasing function. A definition of health in a geriatric person, therefore, must be based on ability to function rather than on perfection of function.

Also, signs, degrees, and rates of aging differ from one person to another person and from one part of the same body to another part. One man may develop many wrinkles and be bald at 40, while another may have few wrinkles and a full head of gray hair at 70. A person of 50 may have the stomach of a 40-year-old, the heart of a 60-year-old, and the liver of an 80-year-old. Nearly every old person has one or more chronic health problems.

Then, too, it is important to remember that signs of aging are seldom sudden or dramatic. In fact, they develop so slowly that, unless deliberately sought, they can be overlooked. Early notice of a sign of aging allows for better treatment and can prevent or slow disability.

It is also important to remember that aging lowers resistance to any illness. A geriatric patient is more prone to acute diseases such as colds, flus, and intestinal infections. Acute disease affects him more severely and he is slower to recover.

In order to observe a geriatric patient, you must do the following:

Be alert to recognize general signs of aging.

Be familiar with the patient's specific history of aging and be alert for changes. (You learn his history from the charge nurse's reports, the patient's health records, staff meetings, and evaluations of the patient.)

Be alert for signs of acute illness.

RECOGNIZING SIGNS OF AGING (10 signs of aging)

Bones grow brittle and break easily. Joints become painful and stiff, restricting motion.

Blood circulation slows. The heart enlarges. Hardening occurs in some blood vessel walls. Clots tend to form in blood vessels. Varicose veins and ulcers are common. Strain on blood vessels causes some to break. High blood pressure or low blood pressure may develop.

Nerves react slower, and the person therefore responds more slowly to any stimulation of the senses. Interests change from active affairs to quieter ones. Trembling may occur. The mind may become easily confused. The person is apt to forget recent happenings and to remember the past with clarity. Speech may become repetitious or difficult.

Teeth may decay and the gums recede and become infected. The desire for food may lessen. Bowel function slows and movements become difficult. Disorders such as diabetes, gallstones, and ulcers may appear. Hemorrhoids may develop. The anus may lose muscle tone and control of bowel function lessen.

Elasticity of the lungs lessens. Breathing may become difficult. Coughing may be frequent. Colds, flus, and upper respiratory infections last longer and require more care.

Kidneys may not function well. The bladder sphincter muscle may lose control and the person may need to urinate often or may dribble urine. Bladder infections may occur.

Sexual interest decreases. The male may develop prostate trouble that can interfere with his ability to void. Glandular slowdown causes figure changes and can trigger depression.

The skin loses elasticity and dries, bruises, wrinkles, infects easily, and heals slowly. Pressure sores or decubitus ulcers easily develop.

Hair thins, dries, and turns gray.
Hearing ability lessens.
The sight blurs, or becomes restricted. Cataracts may form and glaucoma may develop.
Rest and sleep requirements change. The person may need to rest more often after less exertion. He may sleep for shorter periods but need frequent naps.

SYMPTOMS

A healthy body looks, acts, and behaves in certain expected normal ways. When sickness and aging occur, some of these ways change. Any sign of change away from or back toward normal is called a symptom.

When symptoms are confined to a small area of the body, they are called local symptoms.

Example: When skin breakdown occurs, it first shows as a reddened area.

When symptoms occur not only in the local area, but throughout the body, they are called general symptoms.

Example: A person with pneumonia would have local symptoms of cough, chest pain, difficulty in breathing, and bloody discharge from the lungs.

He would have general symptoms of an elevated TPR, a feeling of extreme tiredness or collapse, changes in the color and the degree of dampness of his skin, and changes in the balance of food and fluid intake and waste outputs.

The degree and amounts of these changes would vary from time to time.
So the date and the hour are as necessary to record as the listing of symptoms.
In order to diagnose and treat an illness, a doctor must know the exact location of any symptom and have a clear description of it.

Example: Do not report that "the patient has a pain in his leg."
Report in detail:
Example: "The patient has a throbbing pain in the inner side of his upper left calf. An area about the size of an orange appears somewhat swollen and is reddened. At the center of this area is a small opening in the skin, crusted with dried blood."

Example: Do not say, "The patient has a cold." Do say, "The patient is sneezing. His nose is running, his eyes are watering, and he has a frequent wet cough."

Learn to observe and report by using all of your senses to notice changes in a patient.

See and describe:

The general activity of a patient
Body positionings
Skin textures
Skin color changes
The presence of discharges from any part of the body and the nature of the body's wastes
　　The substance
　　The amount
　　The color
　　The consistency

The smell
The frequency
Facial expressions
Eye expressions
Eye changes

Hear and describe:

How the patient talks
What the patient says
How he reacts to questions
What he leaves unsaid but indicates by actions
Noises that his body makes

Smell and describe:

Any part of the body or discharge

Touch and describe:

Any part of the body
How the patient's body reacts to your touch

Get your patient to tell you:

How he sees
How he hears
How his mouth tastes
How he feels
About any pain, note the following:
 The exact location
 The kind of pain
 When it occurs
 How long it lasts
 Does anything relieve it
About his mental condition through conversation and other things.

Bath time offers an excellent chance to observe a patient.

Sometimes there is a sudden onset of alarming symptoms that indicate the patient is in great distress. It is important at these times not to panic. Do what you can for the patient in a calm, reassuring way. Get the charge nurse or doctor at once. Your behavior in such an emergency can mean life or death for your patient. In any event, a calm attitude can control the patient's fear and make the situation easier for him.

VITAL SIGNS

Temperature, pulse, respirations, and blood pressure are called vital signs or signs of life.

About Temperature

Taking the body temperature is an excellent way to help determine how ill the body is. Taking and recording the body temperature at certain hours over a period of time is an excellent way of determining the course of an illness.

On each floor or ward of an institution a small notebook is used to list the name and the times at which each patient should have his temperature taken. This notebook is usually labelled TPR or *Temp*. A temperature is entered in this book next to the name of the patient and also the time at which the temperature was taken. Pulse and respiration counts are always taken at the same time as a temperature and these are also written into the TPR book: temperature first — then pulse — then respirations. Later these readings are recorded in each patient's chart.

Temperature can be taken by using a thermometer in three ways:

Oral (by mouth)

Rectal (inserted into the anus)

Axillary (under the armpit)

Oral Temperature

The glass oral thermometer has a long slender tip. This tip is placed under the tongue and the lips are closed tightly around the thermometer. It is left in place for 3 minutes. The normal temperature by mouth is 98^6. An oral or axillary temperature is always taken when the rectal area is sensitive.

Rectal Temperature

The glass rectal thermometer has a fat or bulb-shaped silver tip. Lubricant is put on the tip and it is inserted into the anus (the opening of the rectum) for a distance of about 3 inches. It is left in place for 3 minutes. Normal rectal temperature is 99^6. A rectal or axillary temperature is always taken when there is any interference with a person's ability to breathe and when a patient is confused. When used on a geriatric patient, a rectal thermometer should always be inserted and held by you during the entire time it is in place. Insert gently, never force; rotate or change direction of insertion if resistance is met.

Axillary Temperature

Either an oral or a rectal thermometer may be used to take an axillary temperature. The silver tip is placed well inside the armpit, and the arm is held tight against the body. The thermometer is left in place for 10 minutes. Normal axillary temperature is 97^6. An axillary temperature may be taken if neither an oral nor a rectal temperature can be taken. (*Example:* On a patient who cannot close his mouth and who has hemorrhoids.)

About Glass Thermometers

A small wad of cotton should be placed at the bottom of the thermometer container to prevent breaking or chipping the thermometer.

The container should always be filled with sterilizing solution.

Never wash a thermometer in warm or hot water.

When shaking a thermometer, stand clear of nearby objects.

If a thermometer were to break in a patient's mouth:

Tell the patient not to swallow.

Get him to spit out what he can.

Let him rinse his mouth and spit several times.

Examine his mouth for glass bits or cuts.

Report the accident to the supervisor at once.

Bread may be given in an emergency if the patient has swallowed glass. Bread collects the glass bits and lessens the chances of injury.

Taking the Temperature of a Geriatric Patient

The rules for when temperatures of geriatric patients should be taken differ from one nursing home to another and from one level of nursing care to another.

Under normal circumstances, a geriatric resident on a minimal care level seldom requires his temperature to be taken more often than once a week. A resident on a constant medical supervision level may need a daily or more frequent reading. A patient on an acute care level may require a reading every 4 hours. Any patient with an elevated temperature should have frequent temperature checks. Any patient who complains of feeling unusually ill should have an immediate temperature check.

Aging interferes with the body's ability to regulate its temperature. Thermometer readings of geriatric patients often register lower than the normal that is marked on the thermometer. This is not usually a cause for concern. Any reading lower than 97° by mouth, 98° by rectum, and 96° by axilla, however, should be reported to the charge nurse.

Taking a Temperature with a Glass Thermometer

YOU NEED

TPR book

thermometer in a container of sterilizing solution

tissue wipe

lubricant, if rectal thermometer

wristwatch with a second hand

YOU DO THIS

Remove the thermometer from its container of sterilizing solution.

Wipe it with a tissue.

Check the reading, shake and recheck until the reading is below 96.

Insert the thermometer.

Notice the time.

Count the pulse and respirations.

Record the pulse and respirations in the TPR book.

After 3 minutes (or 10 for axillary) remove the thermometer.

Wipe it with a tissue, read, and record the temperature in the TPR book.

Shake down the thermometer and return it to its container of sterilizing solution.

Electric Skin Thermometer

Many nursing homes and hospitals use electric skin thermometers rather than glass mercury-filled ones. The skin thermometer is operated by a battery inside a box that can be held by one hand (Fig. 25). A plastic disposable sheath is put on a rectal or oral probe, and the sheathed probe presented to the patient in the same way as a glass thermometer. The skin thermometer registers accurate temperature on a large, easily read dial within 15 seconds. The sheath is changed before use by another patient. This thermometer is therefore more sanitary, safer, more comfortable, and takes less time than does the glass one.

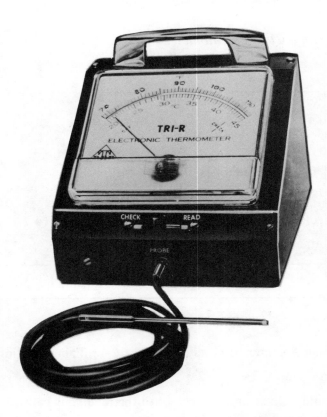

Figure 25. A battery operated thermometer without sheath. (Reprinted by permission of © J. A. Preston Corp., 1971.)

Disposable Oral Thermometer

This thermometer is a short, thin, plastic-coated strip of aluminum. One end of the thermometer has a printed series of numbers ranging from 96–104°F. A row of small dots appears after each number.

MEETING YOUR GERIATRIC PATIENT'S NEEDS

Each of these dots represents two-tenths of a degree ranging from 0.0 to 0.8. Both numbers and dots can be seen easily. Ten or twenty thermometers are supplied in a single package.

To use the thermometer, it must be correctly pulled from the package. Correct pulling activates chemicals in the dots.

The thermometer is placed in the mouth for 30 seconds.

When the thermometer is removed, the patient's temperature is shown by changes in the color of some of the dots. All the dots below the temperature reading turn blue. (*Example:* If the patient's temperature is 98[6], all the dots following the numbers 96 and 97 will change color, and the first three dots following the number 98 will also change color.)

Counting the Pulse

Place the tips of three of your middle fingers along the inside of the patient's wrist starting at the base of the thumb. Roll your fingers over that area until you feel the pulse beat.

Use a watch with a second hand. Start counting the pulse beat when the second hand reaches 12. Count the beat for a full minute or until the second hand returns to 12.

Record the pulse count in the TPR book.

Counting Respirations

Place the patient's wrist so that it rests on his chest. Hold the wrist of the patient as though you were taking his pulse but release the pressure of your fingers so as not to feel the pulse. Watch the patient's chest out of the corner of your eye.

Glance at the second hand of your watch. When that hand reaches 12, count as you feel each rise of the patient's chest. Count the rises for a full minute or until the second hand returns to 12.

Record the respiration count along with the pulse in the TPR book.

Charting Temperature, Pulse, and Respirations

Temperature, pulse, and respirations are recorded on a special sheet of the patient's chart. This sheet is called a graphic sheet because the rise and fall of temperature and pulse are shown by line drawings. It is possible to glance at such a sheet and immediately see the paths of a patient's temperature and pulse rate over a given time.

Although graphic sheets vary from one hospital or nursing home to another, the principle of line drawings is always the same.

Many institutions use blue ink to indicate temperature readings and red ink to show pulse counts. Different dots are used to indicate temperature and pulse. A closed dot may be used for temperature and an open one for pulse.

About Blood Pressure (BP)

Using a Sphygmomanometer, or Blood Pressure Machine

YOU NEED

a stethoscope (a listening aid that magnifies sound)

a sphygmomanometer (a blood pressure machine)

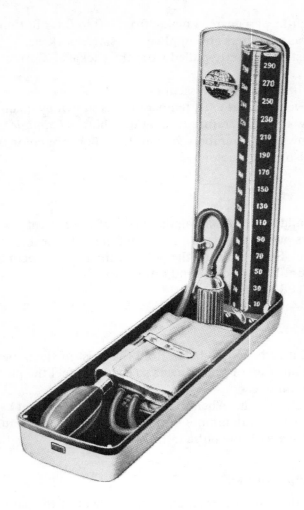

Figure 26. A sphygmomanometer, or blood pressure machine. (Reprinted by permission of © J. A. Preston Corp., 1971.)

YOU DO THIS

Place the patient's arm, palm up, in a natural position. Unless indicated by the doctor, either arm may be used. However, repeated blood pressures should be taken on the same arm.

Wrap the collapsed cuff of the sphygmomanometer around the upper arm just above the elbow and place the arm so that the inner side of the elbow is exposed.

Be sure the cuff tube is attached to the dial tube.

Open the air lock on the bulb.

Find the patient's pulse just below the thumb of the same arm and keep your fingers on the pulse.

MEETING YOUR GERIATRIC PATIENT'S NEEDS

Pump the bulb to fill the cuff with air. Fill until the pulse can no longer be felt. Filling the cuff forces the mercury or dial reading to rise.

Lock the air inlet and let go of the pulse.

Place your stethoscope in position. Be sure the cone or disc sound lock is open. Ear pieces go inside your ears. Press the cone or disc to the inner angle of the elbow below the cuff.

Watch the dial or meter.

Release the air lock as slowly as you can, so that the mercury or dial slowly drops.

Systolic: Listen for the first sound of a beat. Read the number on the dial or column where that sound is first heard.

Diastolic: Continue to listen until the last beat is heard. Read the number on the dial or column where the last beat is heard.

Release all air from the cuff.

Remove the cuff from the patient and write down the two readings in this manner.

B/P <u>120</u> the top reading is the systolic
      80 the lower reading is the diastolic

A blood pressure reading is always charted.

TUBES, TUBING, AND OTHER EQUIPMENT USED IN TREATMENTS

Tubes made of rubber or plastic are important in the treatment of many patients. They are put into natural and surgical body openings in order to drain, give medication to, or wash out a part of the body. Such tubes have special names related to their sizes and specific uses. Many of these tubes are disposable; some are not.

Aides may insert the following tubes:

A *rectal tube* is a thick tube with several large holes at the insertion end and is put through the anus into the rectum for the purpose of letting flatus (gas) out of the intestine. It is inserted in the same way and for the same distance as an enema tube. The open end of a rectal tube is attached to a plastic disposable bag by a rubber band. This prevents tubal leakage from soiling the bed.

An *enema tube* is a rectal tube inserted for the purpose of giving fluids to stimulate bowel action, or giving medication or food. The tube is connected by tubing to a container of fluid hung on a standard. (*See* "Giving Enemas" Your Geriatric Patient Needs Bowel and Bladder Control.)

A *douche nozzle* is a short, hard tube inserted into the vagina to irrigate it (wash it out) or to give medication. The nozzle connects by tubing to a container of fluid hung on a standard.

General Rules for Inserting Tubes

Free the tube of air when giving an enema or douche.
Lubricate the insertion end.
Insert gently, never force.

General Rules for Watching Tubes and Tubing

See that there is no blockage in the tube or tubing. (When blockage occurs, the tube may require irrigation. This is usually done using a sterile bulb syringe, a sterile container, and sterile solution such as normal saline. This equipment is set up at the bedside and kept covered when not in use. Irrigation of tubing should be done only by a professional nurse or under the supervision of a professional nurse.)

See that there are no leaks in the tube or tubing.

See that there is no pull on the tube or tubing.

See that the fluid flows at the rate ordered.

Cleaning and Sterilizing Tubes and Connective Tubing

Most insertion tubes and tubing used in hospitals are disposable. They are used only once. Most come packaged in sterile containers.

No tube or tubing should be thrown away unless its wrapper reads *disposable.*

Tubes that are not disposable must be sterilized between use on patients.

First wash each tube under running cold water and swab the inside, if necessary, to free sticking particles, then sterilize.

APPLYING HEAT AND COLD

Heat and cold treatments can be given internally by food, drink, enema, or irrigation for example, or externally by application to the outer body.

Wherever heat is given, it expands the blood vessels and increases the circulation to that area. So, it is useful in bringing small infections to drain, and in reducing congestion or inflammation. Heat soothes nerve endings and relieves certain pain. It helps relax muscle tension. External heat is given in three ways.

Dry heat is given by lamps, exposure to sunlight, electric pads and blankets, room heating, and hot water bottles.

Moist heat is given by soaks, compresses, steam inhalations, irrigations, baths, and chemical packs.

Medicinal heat is given by applying an irritant, such as oil of wintergreen, liniment, or mustard plaster to the skin.

Cold contracts the blood vessels, decreases the circulation, and deadens nerve endings. It is used to control major infections, such as appendicitis, and to deaden pain. There are three ways to apply external cold.

Dry cold is given by ice caps, air conditioning, and chemical packs.

Moist cold is given by soaks, compresses, baths, and irrigations.

Medicinal cold is sprayed on the skin. Cold is often applied in this fashion to anesthetize a small area for a short time.

Applying Heat or Cold to a Geriatric Patient

It is very important to remember that applying heat or cold to a geriatric patient can be dangerous.

Aging decreases a body's adaptability to temperature changes, and a geriatric patient, therefore, is easily chilled.

Aging decreases body reflex responses, consequently a geriatric patient does not withdraw as quickly from danger and may receive a burn before recognizing the sensation of heat.

Aging decreases a mind's ability to judge. A geriatric patient therefore needs protection from danger.

General Rules for Applying Heat or Cold to a Geriatric Patient

Never give applications of heat or cold except on a doctor's order.

Use lower heat temperature than for a younger patient.

Shorten the length of the treatment.

Use moist heat instead of dry heat. (*Example:* A hot pack instead of a heating pad.)

Use heating pads or blankets with great care. (Most geriatricians will not allow their use.) When used, they should never be put on high, left on a patient for hours, or left on an unattended patient.

Examine the skin before, during, and after applications of heat or cold. If unusual signs occur, report to the charge nurse before beginning or continuing the treatment.

Give skin care before and after a treatment.

Protect the skin with padding.

Watch the patient during and after heat or cold treatment for signs of chilling.

Hot Water Bags

{Burn may occur from hot or cold}

YOU NEED

hot water bag

cover, or towel to cover bag

bath thermometer

YOU DO THIS

Test the water temperature. It should be 110°F. Do not test the temperature of running water. Draw the water into a container, then test.

Half fill the bag with the tested water. Too much water makes the bag heavy.

Lay the bag flat on the sink or table, use the flat of your hand to press the bag gently until water appears in the neck. This removes air from the bag. Air in the bag makes it hard to manage and interferes with the heat radiation to the body.

Put the stopper on as tightly as possible.

Dry the bag well.

Test for leakage by holding the bag upside down.

Put the bag in a cover or wrap it in a towel. It should never be put directly on the skin as there is danger of burning.

Apply the bag to the proper area.

Remove the bag when the water cools.

Reapply as ordered.

Care of the Bag After Use

Empty the water from the bag.
Hang it upside down to drain.
Leave the stopper off.
To store the bag, inflate it with air and put the stopper on. Lightly powder the outer surface of the bag.

Hot Soaks

The immersion of a limb or other part of the body into hot, plain or medicated water is called a hot soak. A doctor might order a hot soak to relieve muscle strain or tension or to localize an infection.

Hydrocollator Steam Pack

A hydrocollator steam pack is a closed fabric envelope that contains a substance that absorbs a great amount of water and retains heat for long time periods. It is ideal for applying moist heat. No wringing is necessary and little dripping occurs. Packs are available in several sizes and are designed to fit body curves (Fig. 27). They can be used over and over again.

Packs are heated by immersion in water at a temperature of 110–120°F. In geriatric facilities, a special electrically heated cabinet that automatically maintains water at the correct treatment temperature is used. This hydrocollator has racks to hold all packs that are not in use.

A pack must be covered with six layers of toweling before it is applied. Special six-layered hydrocollator covers are available and convenient. If a patient has thin, tender, or reddened skin, additional padding should be placed between the skin and the pack. Covers should be washed frequently. If more than one patient uses packs, mark a few covers with each patient's name so that covers can be used for more than one heat application to that patient.

Applying a Hydrocollator Steam Pack

YOU NEED

    steam pack

    six-layered cover

    1 bath towel

    skin lotion

YOU DO THIS

    Check temperature of hydrocollator water.

    Remove correct size pack from hydrocollator.

    Place pack inside six-layered cover.

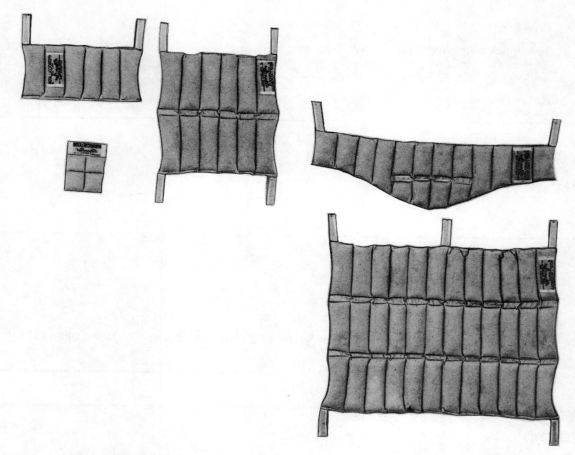

Figure 27. Hydrocollator pads. (Reprinted by permission of © J. A. Preston Corp., 1971.)

Place pack on folded bath towel.

Take pack to bedside.

Position patient comfortably for best application of pack.

Place pack with six-layered cover on correct part of the body.

Hang bath towel over bedside chair or foot of bed.

Leave pack in position on patient for 20–30 minutes. Check the skin for irritation during first few minutes after application.

Remove pack and place on folded towel.

Place both on bedside chair seat or bedside stand.

Give skin care.

Reposition patient.

Adjust bed clothes.

Take pack and cover back to hydrocollator machine.

Remove cover and place on drying rack.

Return the steam pack to hydrocollator rack.

Ice Bags (Caps or Collars)

YOU NEED

ice bag

cover for bag

ice chips. (It is easy to chip ice cubes by jabbing them with the point of an open safety pin.)

YOU DO THIS

Fill the bag half full of ice chips. More than half full makes the bag too heavy.

Squeeze the rest of the bag to expel air.

Screw on the cap.

Test for leakage.

Dry the bag well.

Put on the ice bag cover. Do not apply a bag without a cover.

Apply to the area to be treated.

Remove when ice has melted.

Reapply as directed.

Care of the Ice Bag After Use

Remove the soiled cover and put it in the laundry.
Take off the cap.
Drain the bag and hang it upside down to dry.
To store: Inflate the bag with air. Screw on the cap. Store in a cool, dry place.

MEETING YOUR GERIATRIC PATIENT'S NEEDS

Cold Compresses

YOU NEED

tray

a large basin half filled with crushed ice (Ice is never put directly into compress or soak solution, since a particle of ice can stick to the compress and get onto the skin.)

a smaller basin with the ordered solution

protective pad

towel

rubber gloves, if needed

gauze compresses (a large pile)

paper disposable bag

YOU DO THIS

Follow the general rules for all treatments.

Place the protective pad under the area to be treated.

Cover the pad with the towel.

Position the area to be treated on the towel.

Put on gloves.

Put the gauze compresses into the solution.

Wring out some of the compresses as dry as possible.

Stretch and place them on the area to be treated.

Remove them after a few minutes and discard them into the paper disposable bag.

Use new compresses and repeat the treatment until the time is up. (If there is no drainage, the same compresses can be reused.)

YOU REPORT FOR CHARTING

As for hot compresses.

CHANGING A DRESSING

Sterile dressings should be changed by a doctor or professional nurse unless specific instruction and supervision are given by a doctor or nurse during the changing. However, there are many kinds of unsterile dressings, such as those for colostomy or hemorrhoids, that you will be allowed to change.

YOU NEED

    protective underpad

    disposable bag (usually plastic)

    disposable gloves

    clean dressings

    gauze squares

    basin of warm water

    liquid soap

    salve or ointment if ordered

    a clean binder or tape to hold the dressings in place

YOU DO THIS

    Protect the bed with the underpad.

    Put on the disposable gloves. This protects you from possible contact with germs.

    Remove the old dressings and put them in the disposable bag. This prevents the possible spread of germs.

    Use the gauze squares, warm water, and liquid soap to clean the area.

    Apply salve to the area, if ordered.

    Put on the clean dressings.

    Fasten them with tape or put on a binder.

YOU REPORT FOR CHARTING

    The time of the dressing.

    A description of the drainage on the dressings that you removed.

    A description of the body area from which they were removed.

    The name of any salve applied.

APPLYING AN ELASTIC BANDAGE

An elasticised pressure bandage is often used for the following:

To hold a dressing in place

To support an injured limb

To prevent an injured limb from swelling

To prevent swelling of the feet and legs in patients with heart and kidney diseases

To prevent clots from forming in the leg veins after surgery

To relieve pressure on varicose veins

The bandages are available in hospitals and drug stores. They can be bought without prescription and come in widths of 2, 3, and 4 inches. The width used is determined by the size of the part to be wrapped. An elastic bandage should not be used on a geriatric patient unless ordered by a doctor.

General Rules for Applying an Elastic Bandage

Elevate the part to be bandaged; this lessens blood flow to the part.

Apply the bandage with a gentle, equalized tension and overlapping layers. Ask the patient if the bandage feels tight. It should feel comfortable but give support.

After a bandage is applied, watch for swelling and cold or blue skin below the wrapped area. These signs mean circulation interference, and in that event the bandage should be removed and the condition reported at once.

Remove the bandage at least once in every eight hours and leave it off for 20 minutes before reapplying. The skin should be carefully examined during these rest periods. Changes in the skin should be reported and skin care given before the bandage is replaced. Continuous use of the bandage can cause skin breakdown.

Wash the bandage often and dry it, without stretching, to renew the elasticity. Use a mild suds and rinse well. Geriatric patients often use elastic stockings rather than bandages. These should be cared for in the same way.

Applying an Elastic Bandage to an Ankle

YOU DO THIS

Place the end of the rolled bandage on top of the arch of the foot. Leave the toes exposed.

Wrap the arch twice in the same place to anchor the bandage.

Then wind the bandage around the ankle, back down to the foot, across the arch, and under the foot in a figure eight.

Repeat the figure eight, covering a new area of skin but overlapping the first figure eight. The heel is not wrapped unless so ordered.

Repeat the figure eight if necessary. Then continue wrapping the ankle and leg in spiral fashion, with each turn overlapping the last.

Adjust bandage so that the end of the last turn is on the outside of the leg.

Fasten the bandage with clips or safety pins. The bandage clips are placed on the outside of the leg so that they cannot catch on the other leg.

YOU NEED

Clean elastic stocking

YOU DO THIS

Be sure the stocking is the right size for the patient.

Examine the stocking for holes. Do not use if a hole is present.

Test the stretch of the stocking for elasticity. Do not use it if the stretch is loose, or if it does not return to its original shape after being stretched.

Roll the stocking to its toe end.

Elevate the patient's leg.

Put the toe of the stocking on the patient.

Unroll the stocking to cover the foot and heel.

Smooth the stocking foot so it is free of wrinkles.

Unroll the stocking to the knee.

Smooth the stocking leg so it is free of wrinkles.

Unroll the stocking over the knee and thigh.

Smooth the stocking top so it is free of wrinkles.

Attach the top of the stocking to the girdle or garter belt. (Never use a round leg garter on a geriatric patient. It interferes with the blood supply in the legs.)

PUTTING ON AN ARM SLING

Many commercial styles of arm slings are available and are often used. Read and follow package instructions.

An arm sling is always ordered by the doctor, except for temporary emergency treatment. A triangle of heavy muslin makes a good sling. (Fig. 28)

YOU NEED

triangle of heavy muslin

2 safety pins

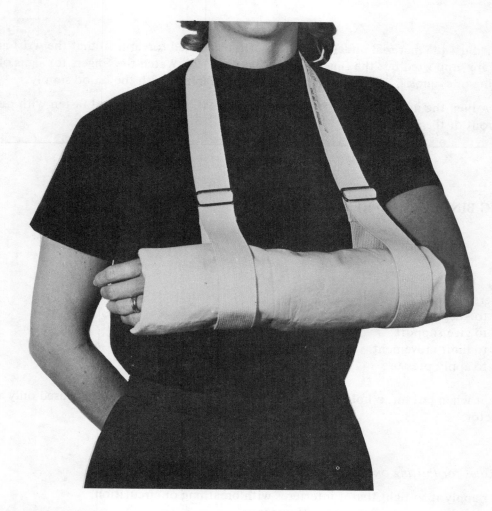

Figure 28.   An arm sling. (Reprinted by permission of © J. T. Posey Co.)

Adjust the material under the length of the affected forearm so that the wrist and the hand are supported but the fingers are free and visible. Watch the fingers for signs of swelling or cyanosis. These signs indicate an interference with the blood supply.

Adjust the material at the elbow to form a neat, snug corner and fasten with pins to the front of the sling.

APPLYING BINDERS AND RESTRAINTS

Binders

Binders are used:
    to keep dressings in place
    to give support
    to limit movement
    to apply pressure

Except when put on to hold dressings in place, binders and restraints are used only when ordered by the doctor.

General Rules for Putting on Any Binder

Never apply it so tight that it interferes with breathing or circulation.
Be sure it is firm enough to serve its purpose.
Be sure it is smooth and without wrinkles.
Be sure any dressing beneath the binder is in the right position.
Be careful when pinning a binder not to stick the patient.

A Scultetus or Many-Tailed Binder

YOU DO THIS

Position the bed flat.

Turn the patient on his side.

Fold the binder in half so that the insides are together.

Place the fold against the patient's back.

Roll the top half of the binder against the patient's back.

MEETING YOUR GERIATRIC PATIENT'S NEEDS

Roll the patient onto his back and, if necessary, onto his other side to release the rolled binder half.

Adjust the tails straight and free of wrinkles.

Apply straps: alternating left and right straps, placing each on an angle across the abdomen, with each strap covering half of the previous strap from the same side. Pull each strap firm and tight. Apply the last two straps in a straight line across the abdomen. Pin on each side. On a geriatric patient, this binder is applied beginning at the pubic area and working upward.

T-Strap Binders

T-strap binders are often used to hold dressings in place on geriatric patients with rectal or urinal leaking. The binders are made of heavy muslin and are easy to launder. There are two types, a single strap and a double strap. The single strap type is used on females, and the double strap type on males. Disposable binders are available.

Applying a T-Strap Binder

YOU NEED

the right binder

2 safety pins

gauze dressing or genital pads

a paper or plastic disposal bag

YOU DO THIS

Remove soiled binder

Remove soiled dressings and put them in the disposal bag.

Place the belt of the binder around the waist with the strap in the center of the back.

Position the dressing or genital pad.

Bring the strap or straps between the thighs and over the dressing.

Use two pins to secure the strap or straps to the belt.

Bed Restraints (Wrist and Ankle)

Restraints (Fig. 29) are used only when a doctor orders them, except when the patient is in danger of harming himself or others. Then, restraints may be put on until the doctor is notified of the patient's condition.

Remember: If one wrist is restrained, the other must also be restrained.

If feet are restrained, wrists must also be restrained.

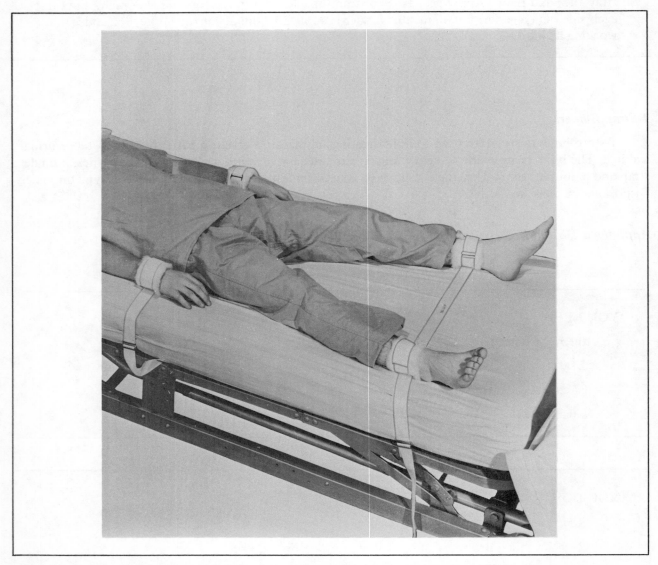

Figure 29. Wrist and ankle restraints. (Reprinted by permission of © J. T. Posey Co.)

Before Applying Bed Restraints

Be sure the patient is in a normal comfortable position.
Bathe the wrists and ankles with warm water.
Dry them well.
Rub them with skin lotion.

Pad them with cotton or foam rubber.

Never fasten restraints so tight that the patient cannot move his limbs.

After Applying Bed Restraints

Watch for skin changes that indicate the blood supply is shut off. White, blue, gray, or cold skin is a sign of poor blood circulation. If such signs occur, remove the restraints.

Check the restraints at regular intervals.

Remove them every 4–6 hours and repeat skin care. Leave off for twenty minutes before reapplying.

Using a Length of Material as a Restraint

Make a restraint knot in the center of the strip of material.

Pad the wrist or foot.

Slip the restraint knot over the padding.

Tighten until secure but not binding. (You should be able to slip two fingers inside the restraint.)

Tie the restraint ends to the frame of the bed, with a square knot.

There are many kinds of restraints in use. Here are some:

A length of quilted material

A length of heavy muslin

A length of heavy cotton tape with attached foam plastic and self-fastening cuffs

Remember: Never use gauze or ropes to restrain a patient. They cut the skin and interfere with circulation.

Many commercial styles of restraints are available and often used. These have the advantages of allowing greater patient comfort and being easier to apply. Some types are disposable. Before applying, read package instructions carefully and then follow them exactly.

Making Knots

Making a Restraint Knot

YOU DO THIS

Place one end of the material on a flat surface while you hold the other.

Make a figure eight next to the end on the flat surface.

Thread the end you hold through the two loops of the figure eight, keeping the other end free.

Adjust the loop to fit the ankle or wrist.

Knot once to fasten.

Tie the ends to the bed with a square knot.

YOU DO THIS

Hold an end in each hand.

Place the right end over the left end and tie. Then place the left end over the right end and tie.

Mitt Restraints

Geriatric patients with mental confusion may pick at bed covers or at their skin until it becomes sore. Mitt restraints prevent self-injury (Fig. 30).

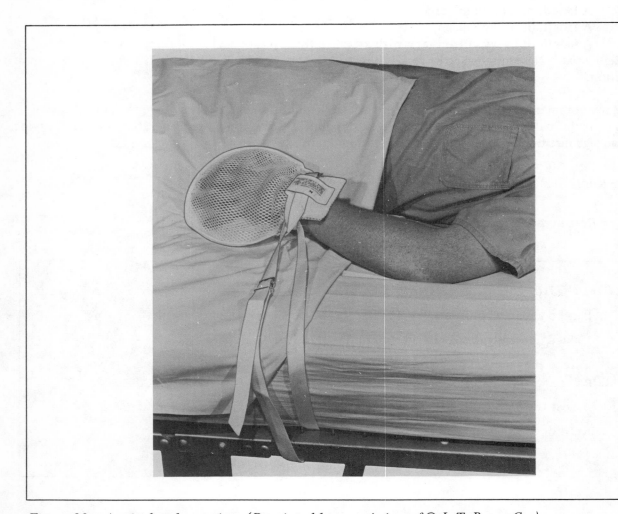

Figure 30. A mitt hand restraint. (Reprinted by permission of © J. T. Posey Co.)

9

YOUR GERIATRIC PATIENT NEEDS FOOD AND FLUID BALANCE

STUDY GUIDE

What six things does a doctor consider before ordering a diet for a geriatric patient?

Why is chronic disease always the first consideration?

What can a patient's blood chemistry indicate to the doctor?

What are the geriatric patient's nutritional needs? How may his diet differ from that of a normal adult?

How can digestive and intestinal function affect the patient's diet?

Why do doctors prefer geriatric patients to stay thin?

Should a geriatric patient always have three big meals a day?

What should you do before a meal is presented to a patient?

What should you do when a meal is presented?

What should you do after a geriatric patient eats?

What should you report to the charge nurse?

What should you do about meals for the patient you care for in a private home?

What does good nutrition do?

What food substances does the human body need?

What four groups of foods furnish the body's daily requirements?

What is meant by dairy foods?

How much of each food group should a geriatric patient eat each day?

What are the best ways to prepare foods?

Why should you save the water in which vegetables have been cooked?

What standard diets are used in the care of the geriatric patient?

How does a full liquid diet differ from a clear liquid diet?

How does a soft diet differ from a bland diet?

141

How do you prepare a helpless patient for feeding?

Tell how to feed liquids to a helpless patient.

How do you feed solids to a helpless patient?

How often should patients receive fresh water?

What should you know before you give a patient drinking water?

What does fluid balance mean?

When does a doctor order intake measured?

What is the normal fluid intake for one day?

What is the normal fluid output?

What does PO mean?

Name things that would be considered PO fluids.

Name things that would be considered IV fluids.

How else might fluid be taken in by a patient?

How do you record the intake of any fluid?

How do you find out the fluid intake for one day?

Where is an intake sheet usually placed?

What should be on the intake sheet to indicate for whom the sheet is intended?

How should you train yourself to use an intake sheet?

What is a premeasured list?

How would you use a premeasured list?

How many cc. are in 1 oz.?

How would you find out how many cc. are in 4 oz.?

How do fluids leave the body?

How would you record sweating or incontinence?

How would you describe vomiting for a chart?

What should be done with drainage fluid?

How do you use an output sheet?

How do you identify an output sheet as belonging to a specific patient?

How can you measure output at home?

How would urine taken by catheterization be measured?

How would you measure the urine of a patient with a Foley catheter or condom drainage?

THE GERIATRIC PATIENT'S DIET

A doctor considers many things before ordering a diet for a geriatric patient. Some of the main considerations are:

Whether the patient has one or more chronic diseases.
The patient's blood chemistry and general health.
The patient's nutritional needs.
The patient's decreased digestive and intestinal function.
The patient's weight.
The patient's eating habits, tastes, and religious restrictions.

Chronic disease is always the first consideration. Diabetes, hypertension (high blood pressure), and many other conditions can be controlled only by special diets.

A patient's blood chemistry reveals much about the health of his body. Abnormal readings on blood tests are causes for a doctor to make adjustments in a patient's diet. For example, if the blood potassium reading were low, a doctor might order a low salt diet and increased intake of specific foods, such as orange juice, that are rich in potassium.

A geriatric patient requires foods from the same basic nutritional groups as any adult. He needs meat or other protein, fruits and vegetables, bread and cereal, and dairy products. As aging decreases his activity, however, he may require decreasing total food intake. He also may need more protein to help repair tissues affected by the increasing cellular destruction of aging, more fruits and vegetables to stimulate bowel function, additional vitamins and minerals in tablet or capsule form, alcohol or coffee for general stimulation, or no coffee or alcohol for decreased stimulation.

Many problems can result from decreased digestive and intestinal function, and the doctor must consider the patient's specific ones. For example, a patient may have ill-fitting false teeth due to gum shrinkage, be unable to digest milk, have a history of diverticulitis (a pocket in the intestinal tract that is subject to frequent infection), and suffer from constipation. For such a patient, the doctor might order a soft diet, limited intake of milk products, no spices or roughage, and daily prune juice.

Most geriatricians agree that an older person should tend to be thin. Excess weight strains the heart and other organs and interferes with physical activity. No caloric restrictions are put on the patient's diet unless he is overweight or gaining weight. Then, the doctor might order a diet with limited intake of fats and carbohydrates (sugars and starches).

As a person grows older, his eating habits sometimes change. He seems to eat less at a meal but to require food more often than three times a day. Doctors recommend frequent, smaller meals — five or six meals instead of three. The person should be able to select foods that he likes whenever they fill his special dietary requirements.

Geriatric Aide's Mealtime Duties

As a geriatric aide working in a nursing home or day care center, your duties at mealtime are as follows:

Before a Meal Is Presented

Tell the patient it is time for the specific meal, that is: breakfast, lunch, tea, dinner, and so forth.
Inquire if the patient needs to use the toilet or commode and help him to do so, if necessary.
See that the patient is positioned comfortably and in the best way for him to eat. When possible, let him eat with others.
See that the patient has his own adaptive feeding devices and is able to use them (Figs. 31 and 32). Check devices for defects.
Protect the patient's clothing with a bib or napkin.

When the Meal Is Presented

Check the meal to see that it is the right one for the patient. (He may be on a special diet.)
Prepare food servings in the best way for the patient to eat. (He may need meat to be cut or bread to be buttered.)

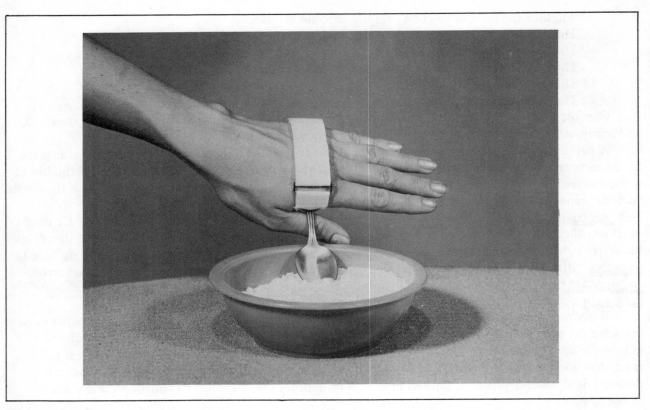

Figure 31. A self-care feeding device. (Reprinted by permission of © J. T. Posey Co.)

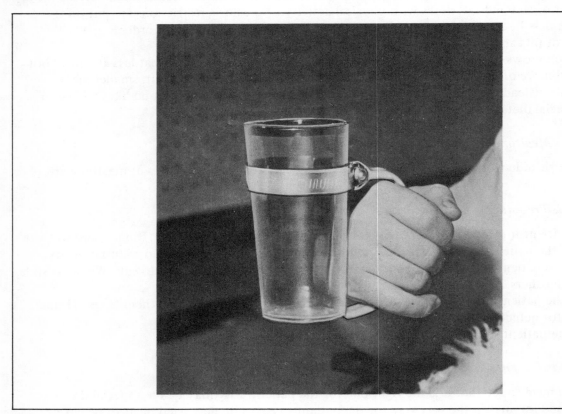

Figure 32. Another device for meals. (Reprinted by permission of © J. A. Preston Corp., 1971.)

MEETING YOUR GERIATRIC PATIENT'S NEEDS

Set the food before the patient so that he has the best access to it.
Encourage the patient to eat.
Observe how he uses adaptive equipment.
Help him to eat when necessary.

After Eating

Remove any adaptive devices and clean them. (These are usually kept in the patient's room and should be marked with the patient's name.)
Check the devices for defects.
Remove the bib or napkin and see that the patient's face and hands are cleaned. (Many facilities use disposable moist towelettes for this purpose and put them next to the patient's place setting at each meal.)
Check the remains of the patient's meal to determine what and how much he has eaten.
Reposition the patient as needed.

Report to the Charge Nurse

any change in the patient's appetite.
any change in the patient's ability to feed himself.
any defect in a feeding device.
any change in the patient's general condition.

Preparing Food for a Geriatric Patient at Home

If you are caring for a geriatric patient at home, your duties include all those already mentioned. In addition, you should know the specific diet that the doctor has ordered for the patient and shop for and prepare the patient's food. Parttime home aides should prepare or arrange for all the patient's daily meals.

Many older people seem to lose their appetites and to become disinterested in food. Many have small incomes. When they must shop for and prepare their own food, eating becomes a function that some are unable or unwilling to perform because of the effort and expense.

National and local governments and charitable organizations are taking an interest in the nutritional welfare of older citizens at home.

Some organizations provide "meals on wheels." These are daily hot meals delivered once daily to older people. Other groups serve inexpensive hot meals to those over 65 in school, church, and social cafeterias. A few restaurants offer "senior citizen specials" or inexpensive daily nonchoice hot meals served during off-rush hours. You should learn what community services are available for older citizens and help your patient to benefit from them when possible.

NUTRITION

Good nutrition means fulfilling the body's needs for certain elements. A proper diet prevents disease, gives energy, aids growth and repair of tissues, regulates the body's elimination, and stimulates appetite. The human body needs different amounts of the following substances:
Proteins to build, repair and maintain tissues.
Carbohydrates to give heat and energy.
Fats to help digestion and give energy.
Vitamins and minerals to maintain proper body functions
Water to maintain healthy fluid balance and aid in discharging wastes.

Necessary foods are divided into four groups, and for good nutrition an aged person should have the following amounts of foods from these groups every day:

1. Dairy foods: two or more glasses of milk.
   Cheese, ice cream, and other milk-made foods can supply part of the milk.
2. Meat: Two or more servings of meat, fish, poultry, eggs, or cheese.
3. Vegetables and fruits: Four or more servings, which should include dark green and yellow vegetables and citrus fruit or tomato.
4. Breads and cereals: Four or more servings.

SELECTING AND PREPARING FOODS

Talk to the patient to learn his likes and dislikes and plan his meals with these in mind.

Appeal to his senses. Select foods that look appetizing, smell good, and have different textures. Select foods that furnish the patient's daily needs.

Cook foods in the simplest way. Bake, broil, boil, or steam them. Cook vegetables quickly in a small amount of water. Save any liquid left in the pot after cooking because it is rich in vitamins and minerals. Use this liquid in soups, in vegetable drinks, or in cooking other foods.

Avoid most fried foods, rich sauces, and heavy desserts. These foods tax digestion, decrease appetite, and do not furnish the best nourishment.

DIETS

Doctors order certain standard diets.

Clear Liquid Diet

Allows: Only clear broths, plain flavored gelatins, clear tea, coffee, and carbonated drinks, such as ginger ale, are given.

Small amounts of fluids are offered about every 2 hours.

Meal Plan for a Clear Liquid Diet:
        8:00 A.M. — coffee or tea
        10:00 A.M. — ginger ale
        12:00 Noon — clear chicken broth, orange gelatin
        2:00 P.M. — tea
        4:00 P.M. — mineral or carbonated water
        6:00 P.M. — beef bouillon, raspberry gelatin
        8:00 P.M. — tea

A geriatric patient might receive a clear liquid diet after a digestive upset.

Full Liquid Diet

Allows: Strained cream soups, thin cooked cereals, strained fruit juices, sherbets or vanilla ice cream, junket, custard, and milk added to the clear liquid diet. Small servings are offered every 2 hours.

Meal Plan for a Full Liquid Diet:
        8:00 A.M. — small glass of strained orange juice, coffee, farina, milk
        10:00 A.M. — beef broth

146

12:00 Noon — strained cream of carrot soup, vanilla ice cream, tea with lemon
2:00 P.M. — apple juice
4:00 P.M. — chicken broth
6:00 P.M. — strained vegetable soup, custard, coffee with milk
8:00 P.M. — gelatin, glass of milk

A geriatric patient might receive a full liquid diet as an in-between diet from clear liquid to soft diet, after dental surgery.

Soft Diet

Allows:
Breads: White, fine whole wheat, and seedless rye breads
Cereals: Dry cereals
Fine white cereals such as farina, Cream of Wheat, cornmeal, rice
Strained coarse cereals such as oatmeal, Wheatena, grits
Crackers: White crackers
Desserts: Custard
Tapioca, rice, and bread pudding
Sponge or angel cake, plain
Frozen and gelatin desserts
Cooked and canned soft fruit without seeds and skin, such as apricots, applesauce, peaches, pears, plums
Ripe bananas, orange and grapefruit sections without membrane
Eggs: (not fried)
Fluids: All drinks (except alcoholic) and strained soups
Meat: Tender meat (ground is best), poultry, fish
Milk and Cheese: Milk, soft cheese, such as cream, cottage, and grated American in a sauce
Pasta: Plain noodles, spaghetti, and macaroni
Vegetables: Cooked asparagus, beets, carrots, peas, spinach, string beans, squash without seeds, mashed sweet potato
White potato without skin, prepared any way except fried.
Avoid: Coarse dark breads, whole-grain crackers, coarse dark cereals
Rich pastries and any dessert with nuts, coconut, or fruits not on the allowed list
Raw fruit except juice, ripe banana, orange and grapefruit sections
Tough meat, gristle and meat fat, salted or smoked meat and fish
Spicy seasonings
Raw, coarse, and strong-flavored vegetables

Meal Plan for Soft Diet:
Breakfast:
Soft fruit or fruit juice
Cereal with milk
Egg
Toast
Butter or fortified margarine
Coffee or tea

Luncheon or supper:
Choice of soft cheese, tender meat, fish, poultry, or egg
Potato or substitute

Cooked vegetable
Bread
Butter or margarine
Fruit
Milk

Dinner:
Tomato, orange or grapefruit juice
Tender meat, fish, or fowl
Potato
Cooked vegetable
Bread
Butter or margarine
Dessert
Milk

Between-meal nourishment: Milk, cocoa, fruit juice
A geriatric patient might receive a soft diet if he is unable to chew, swallow, or digest a regular diet.

Bland Diet

This is the same as a soft diet but without seasonings, stimulants, or roughage. It is often given in frequent small feedings rather than meals.

Meal Plan for a Bland Diet:
Amounts should be about half average size.
8:00 A.M. — strained orange juice or applesauce
Puffed Rice or farina with milk
decaffeinated coffee
10:00 A.M. — beef bouillon
white soda cracker
12:00 Noon — strained tomato or apricot juice
poached egg or lean broiled ground meat
mashed or baked potato without skin
3:00 P.M. — tea with lemon or milk
ladyfinger
6:00 P.M. — broiled fish or breast of chicken
creamed spinach or carrot puree
gelatin salad with peeled canned fruit and cottage cheese
decaffeinated coffee
8:00 P.M. — baked custard or rice pudding

A geriatric patient might receive a bland diet for disorders of the stomach or intestines.

Regular Diet

Meal Plan for a Full, Regular, or Normal Diet:
Breakfast:
Citrus fruit or juice
Whole-grain or enriched cereal with milk and sugar
Egg

Whole wheat toast
Butter or margarine
Coffee, tea, or cocoa with cream and sugar

Luncheon or supper:
Cheese, meat, fish, or eggs
Potato or substitute
Vegetable
Salad with dressing
Whole wheat or enriched bread
Butter or margarine
Fruit (stewed or fresh)
Milk
Tea or coffee

Dinner:
Soup, fruit or juice
Meat, fish, or fowl
Potato or substitute
Vegetable
Whole wheat or enriched bread
Butter or margarine
Dessert
Milk
Tea or coffee

Bedtime feeding:
Milk, cocoa, or fruit juice may be given if the patient is hungry.

A geriatric patient would receive a regular diet if there were nothing in his condition to contraindicate it.

Feeding a Helpless Patient

Stand or sit beside the patient.
Take as much time as necessary and have a relaxed, pleasant attitude.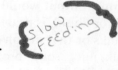
Encourage the patient to communicate his likes and dislikes.
Place a napkin or towel under the patient's chin.

Giving Liquids

Do not fill the glass or cup. Be sure the liquid is not too hot or too cold. Place one of your hands under the patient's pillow to raise his head if necessary. Hold the glass or cup in your other hand and let the patient control it.

If the patient cannot raise his head, turn his head toward you. Put a drinking straw into the liquid and insert the straw into the patient's mouth. Tell the patient to draw on the straw.

Giving Solids

Ask the patient if he would like to have the foods on his tray in any special order.
Use a fork or spoon to offer a small serving.
Give the patient time to chew. Be sure the patient swallows one bite before giving another.

Wipe the mouth when necessary.

Notice and report how much of his meal the patient has eaten.

Notice and report if the patient has trouble chewing and swallowing any particular food or type of food.

DRINKING WATER

You may be asked to pass drinking water. Fresh water should be given to all patients who are permitted water at least once on an 8-hour tour of duty. Water pitchers are collected, filled with ice and fresh water, and then redistributed. Clean glasses are usually given out at the same time.

Once in 24 hours, metal pitchers and glasses are sterilized. This is usually done by the aide who works 11:00 P.M. to 7:00 A.M. or 12:00 Midnight to 8:00 A.M.

Things You Should Know Before Giving Any Drinking Water

Know which patients are on measured fluid intake and what amount of water you should give to each of them.

Know which patients are to receive nothing orally, and are not allowed drinking water.

FLUID BALANCE

Fluid balance means that the amount of liquid put out by the body is equal to the amount taken in. Many geriatric conditions can upset this balance.

MEASURING FLUID INTAKE

Restoring or maintaining the balance can be difficult. Then the doctor wants to know exactly how much fluid is taken in and put out by the patient each day.

The average daily fluid intake for the normal adult of medium size is 3 quarts or 3,000 cc.

A normal output would be about 250 cc. (or half a pint) less. That would be 2,750 cc.

Fluid, or liquid, is usually taken in by mouth (PO). PO fluid intake includes anything that the patient drinks or that dissolves to liquid if taken in his mouth. Water, milk, eggnog, milk shake, malted milk, juice, soup, broth, tea, coffee, soda, beer, ice cream, ice, sherbet, junket, and gelatin are all counted as PO fluids.

Sometimes fluid is taken in by vein (IV). Intravenous, or IV fluids, include blood, plasma, normal saline (NS), dextrose water (D/W).

On occasion, fluid intake may result from a retention enema or from fluid injection under the skin.

Regardless of the way it is taken in, a record must be kept of the time, amount, and method of entry of any fluids taken. All IV fluid intake is totaled at the end of each 24 hours. All PO fluid intake is totaled at the end of each 24 hours. All retained rectal fluid intake is totaled at the end of each 24 hours. All skin injection fluid of more than 5 cc. is totaled at the end of each 24-hour period. Then all of these totals are added together to get the patient's fluid intake for that day.

When a patient is on measured intake, an intake sheet and pencil may be taped to the patient's bedside table. The patient's name is always put on the sheet.

Mark down on this sheet the PO fluid and amount taken whenever you remove any glass, pitcher, cup, dish, container, or tray from the bedside of a patient on measured intake.

Premeasured Lists

Many nursing homes and hospitals use special intake sheets which list, at the top or bottom of the page, all of the containers that the institution uses for oral feedings. These may include water pitcher, water glass, juice glass, large glass, coffee cup, individual tea pot, dessert glass, and paper cup. Next to each item listed is the amount of fluid that the container holds when filled.

If the list reads "coffee cup 150 cc.," you would offer your patient a full cup of coffee. If the patient drank only half of the coffee and left the rest, you would mark down on the intake sheet "coffee 75 cc." since that would be half of the listed amount for a full cup.

At the end of each 8-hour shift, amounts marked on the intake sheet are added and that total charted.

At the end of each 24-hour day, the totals given on the three shifts are added together, and that sum charted as the oral fluid intake for that day.

In institutions where premeasured listings are not used, oral fluids are measured in beakers or pitchers marked in cc.

Pour the liquid to be given into the measure. Read the amount in cc. Then put the liquid into a container to offer it to the patient. When the patient has drunk his fill, measure the remaining amount of fluid. Subtract these remaining cc. from the number of cc. offered to the patient. The answer will be the cc. that the patient has taken.

To change ounces into cc., you have only to multiply the number of ounces by the number of cc. in one ounce.

$$1 \text{ oz.} = 30 \text{ cc.}$$
$$4 \text{ oz.} = 120 \text{ cc.}$$

$$\begin{array}{r} 4 \text{ oz.} \\ \times 30 \\ \hline 120 \text{ cc. in 4 oz.} \end{array}$$

MEASURING FLUID OUTPUT

Fluids can leave the body through sweating, vomiting, liquid stools, heavy bleeding, etc. Most fluid leaves the body through urination. Sometimes a patient has a drainage tube inserted into a body opening.

Sweat, liquid stools, and blood loss are difficult to measure, although a descriptive note should be made on the patient's chart if any of these occur.

Example: 2:00 P.M. Perspiring lightly.
4:00 P.M. Sweating heavily. Patient's sheets and gown wet through.
10:00 A.M. Bowel movement. Large amount of dark brown liquid stool.

Vomiting (emesis) can be measured if it is liquid enough and if the patient has vomited into a container. Otherwise it must be estimated.

Example: 1:00 A.M. Emesis of about 180 cc. of partly digested food.
4:00 A.M. Emesis 6 ounces (360 cc.) of yellow liquid.
6:00 A.M. Incontinent of urine. Four bed pads soaked through.

Any drainage from the body through tubes into containers should be measured as needed or every 8 hours and the amount recorded.

Measuring Urine

Hospital or Nursing Home Method

An output sheet that bears the patient's name is put into the utility room or private bathroom. After each voiding the urine is measured in a beaker, or pitcher, marked in cc. The amount of urine and time of voiding are written on the output sheet. At the end of each 8-hour shift, amounts are totaled and charted. At the end of each 24 hours, the totals from the three shifts are added together and charted as the patient's total output for that day.

Home Method

Keep a plastic or glass measuring pitcher marked in ounces in the bathroom. Label the pitcher *Urine Only*. Use this pitcher to measure each voiding. Keep a record of these amounts. Change the amounts measured from oz. into cc. The pitcher should be thrown away when no longer needed by the patient.

Remember:

1 oz. = 30 cc.	6 oz.
6 oz. = 180 cc.	x30 cc.
	180 cc.

Catheterization

Sometimes a patient has urine withdrawn by a catheter, or tube, inserted into the bladder to drain it. This is a procedure that requires sterile technique. If the urine withdrawn by catheterization were needed for a specimen it would be measured in a sterile pitcher and the amount marked down on the output sheet before sending it to the lab. Only professional nurses or doctors should catheterize patients.

Urinary Drainage

Some patients have Foley indwelling catheters or condoms to drain their urine. Such drainage devices empty into disposable plastic bags. Some of these bags have measures marked on them so you can read the amount in the bag before you empty it; if the bag is not marked, the urine in the bag must be emptied into a measuring pitcher. Each time the bag is emptied, the amount is written on the output sheet. You empty these bags as needed and always at the end of each 8-hour shift. (*See* Your Geriatric Patient Needs Bowel and Bladder Control.)

10

YOUR GERIATRIC PATIENT NEEDS SLEEP, REST, POSITIONING, AND TRANSFERRING

STUDY GUIDE

What happens to a person who is deprived of dream sleep?

How many continuous hours of sleep do geriatric patients require?

How do many geriatric patients prepare for sleep?

In addition to night sleep, how much rest does a geriatric patient need?

When a bed patient has problems moving about in bed, what routine should be started?

Give five general rules for handling a geriatric patient.

Give seven general rules for positioning yourself when handling a patient.

Give five general rules for positioning a patient in bed.

How can you prevent the legs of a bed patient from rotating?

Give eight general rules for lifting and moving a bed patient.

Tell how to lift a bed patient to a sitting position.

Tell how to slide a bed patient nearer.

Tell how to pull up a mattress when a patient can help you.

Tell how to pull up a mattress when a patient cannot help you.

Tell how to pull a helpful patient up in bed.

Tell how to pull a helpless patient up in bed.

Tell how to use a drawsheet to roll and lift a patient.

How can you encourage a patient to help himself turn and sit up?

Give six rules for positioning a patient in a chair.

Of what should you be careful when using a chair restraint?

Tell how you transfer a patient from the bed to a wheelchair.

Tell how a patient transfers from bed to wheelchair.

Tell how a patient transfers from wheelchair to straight chair.

Tell how you transfer a helpless patient to a wheelchair.

How is a tilt table used?

When is the blood pressure taken on a patient using a tilt table?

For what should a patient on a tilt table be checked?

Tell how to place a patient on a tilt table.

What is a mechanical lifter?

How can you calm the fears of a patient using a mechanical lifter for the first time?

Tell how to transfer a patient from bed to chair using a mechanical lifter.

When should sling supports be removed from the patient?

What special safety rules protect a patient when using a mechanical lifter?

Tell the role of each person participating in a three-person carry.

SLEEP

In recent years studies have been made of sleep and brain activity during sleep. Researchers have found that in the process of sleeping, the brain goes through several distinct changes in activity. One of these changes is called REM (Rapid Eye Movement) because the eyes jerk restlessly beneath closed lids.

REM sleep is associated with dreaming. Studies show that dreaming is essential for health. Deprived of dream sleep, any person becomes irritable, loses muscle control, and grows mentally confused. During the next dream sleep period, a person will dream more often to make up for lost dreaming time. All people therefore need sufficient dream sleep.

Older people, however, do not seem to require the average eight hours of continuous sleep needed by most younger adults. Geriatric patients may sleep only a few continuous hours, awakening often to urinate, to drink water, to eat snacks, to listen to the radio, to read, etc. Sometimes they seem to awaken only to reassure themselves that they are in familiar surroundings.

Although each geriatric patient's sleeping pattern differs, most have preparatory rituals for sleep. Older people can be very specific in their wants and in the exact placement of things. One might want the shade of a lamp positioned just so, a bedpan or urinal placed on a chair within easy reach, a radio on a special corner of the bedside table, eyeglasses and kleenex positioned just so, an extra pillow, a certain blanket, etc. Sometimes the demands can seem time consuming and unnecessary. However the older person will respond very well to your patience in meeting his demands. He will feel secure and will sleep better.

Rest

Besides night sleep, the geriatric patient usually requires several rest and nap periods during the day. Most geriatricians recommend an hour or two rest period after the midday meal, during which the patient may want to go to bed. Other rest periods should be arranged to suit the patient's need. Many geriatric patients are able to doze while sitting, even in crowded or noisy situations.

When a patient is expected to walk an unusual distance or climb many stairs, a small lightweight chair can be taken along. Then the person can stop for rest periods whenever he feels the need.

MEETING YOUR GERIATRIC PATIENT'S NEEDS

POSITIONING

Aging affects the balance and strength of a geriatric patient. Consequently, he becomes increasingly dependent on your help to position himself in bed or a chair, to lift himself from a lying to a sitting position, and to transfer himself from bed to a chair or wheelchair.

For bed patients who have problems with moving about in bed, a routine of regular turning should be carried out by nursing personnel. Such a routine is usually scheduled every 2 hours during an entire 24-hour day. When possible, a patient is turned from side to back to other side and then onto the stomach. A large part of your duties as a geriatric aide may be the faithful and considerate performance of this duty. (*See* Your Geriatric Patient Needs Skin Care.)

GENERAL RULES FOR HANDLING A GERIATRIC PATIENT

Tell the patient what you intend to do.
Don't place your hands on a pressure area or incision.
If the patient has painful joints, do not take hold of a joint but grasp the arm or leg above or below the joint.
If the patient has painful muscles, do not take hold of the muscles, but grasp the joint.
Whenever possible, get the patient to help you.

GENERAL RULES FOR POSITIONING YOURSELF WHEN HANDLING A PATIENT

Position yourself so as to perform in the best way and prevent injury to your own body.
Wear comfortable, low-heeled shoes.
Stand erect.
Stand as close to your patient as possible.
Stand flat with feet apart.
Point your toes in the direction of movement.
Bend your knees and use arm and thigh muscles rather than back muscles.

POSITIONING YOUR PATIENT IN BED

General Rules

A patient should be positioned on his side, back or stomach, so that his spine is straight, his body relaxed, and his arms and legs flexed (bent). Hips and knees should be extended from time to time to prevent contracture (inability to extend a body part).

A firm mattress and springs maintain the patient's body in good alignment and make it easier to move and turn the patient (Fig. 33). A bedboard may be used if the mattress sags from the weight of the body.

A footboard may be used to position the patient's feet at right angles to the legs and to prevent bedding from drawing tightly over the feet.

Tight bedding must be avoided. It causes not only discomfort, but also in-grown toenails and tightening of the heel cord. When the heel cord tightens, it is impossible for a patient to stand or walk without pain.

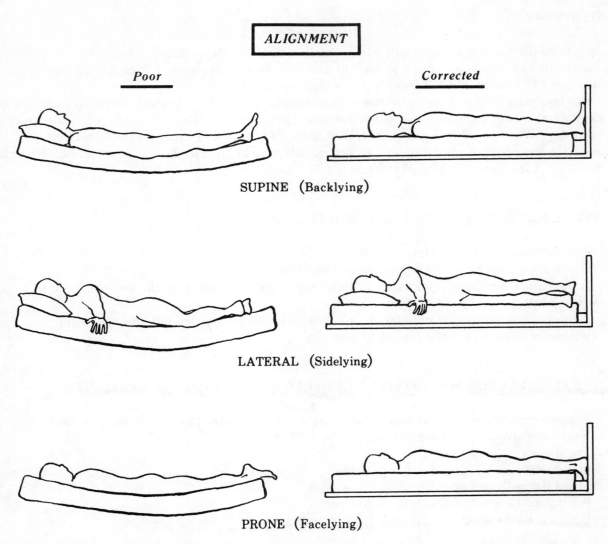

ALIGNMENT

Poor | Corrected

SUPINE (Backlying)

LATERAL (Sidelying)

PRONE (Facelying)

Figure 33. Examples of good and bad body alignment in bed. (Reprinted from Elementary Rehabilitation Nursing Care, U. S. Public Health Service, Division of Nursing.)

Support can be given to hips, knees, shoulder, and other body parts by using pads, pillows, rolled towels, or rolled bath blankets (Fig. 34). These are preferred to rubber rings or doughnuts because they interfere with blood circulation and cause other pressure-sensitive areas. (See Your Geriatric Patient Needs Skin Care.)

Preventing Legs from Rotating

With sandbags:

Sandbags can be placed along the sides of the leg (from hip to knee) to keep the leg from rotating.

With a trochanter roll:

A trochanter roll may be used to prevent legs from rotating outward (Fig. 34).

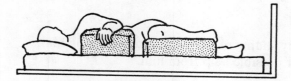

Pillows supporting upper arm and leg
in good alignment

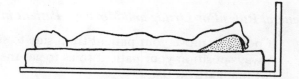

Pillow used to keep good foot alignment
and also relax knees by slight flexing

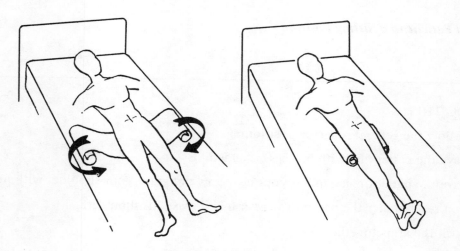

Trochanter Roll

Figure 34. Examples of positioning with support. (Reprinted from Elementary Rehabilitation Nursing Care, *U.S. Public Health Service, Division of Nursing.)*

Making A Trochanter Roll

YOU NEED

a sheet or bath blanket

YOU DO THIS

Fold the sheet in quarters lengthwise.

Place it crosswise under the patient, centering it at his hip.

Roll each side of the sheet under until it rests firmly against the thigh.

Tuck the roll slightly under the thigh.

General Rules For Lifting and Moving a Patient in Bed

If possible, move your patient from side to side by sliding or rolling instead of lifting him.

Always position your patient so as to get the best possible help from him.

Put the mattress flat.

Remove any pillows.

Position the patient on his back and as close to you as possible.

Raise his knees so that the bottom of his feet are slightly apart and rest flat on the bed.

Bend your knees and hips, and use your thigh and arm muscles rather than your back.

Always get help if the patient is heavy.

Lifting a Bed Patient to a Sitting Position

YOU DO THIS

Follow the general rules for positioning.

Have the patient lie with his legs extended.

Have the patient reach under your near arm and grasp your shoulder with his near hand.

You reach under the patient's near arm and grasp his shoulder.

Lock the arms together.

Bend and then reach your arm under the patient's head and shoulders so that his head rests on your forearm and your hand grasps his far shoulder.

Avoid breathing in the patient's face.

Pull back to lift the patient.

Sliding a Bed Patient Nearer

YOU DO THIS

Follow the general rules for lifting and moving.

Hold your hands palms up and close together.

Slip both of your hands well underneath both of your patient's legs just below his knees.

Pull the legs toward you. Then, holding your hands in the same way, slip them well under the patient's hips.

Pull the hips toward you.

Then, slip your near arm under the patient's shoulders so that his head rests on your forearm and you grasp his far shoulder with your hand.

Grasp his near shoulder with your other hand and pull toward you.

Pulling Up the Mattress When Your Patient Is Able to Help

YOU DO THIS

Follow the general rules for lifting and moving.

Have the patient grasp the head of the bed by lifting his arms over his head.

Stand at one side of the bed and half-facing the head.

Bend your knees.

Take hold of the mattress loops.

On the count of three, you and the patient pull together.

Pulling Up the Mattress When Your Patient Is Unable to Help

YOU DO THIS

Follow the general rules for lifting and moving.

Two people stand one on either side of the bed.

Both take hold of mattress loops.

They pull together on the count of three.

Pulling Your Patient Up in Bed

YOU DO THIS

Follow the general rules for lifting and moving.

Have the patient bend his knees and dig the soles of his feet against the mattress.

Place your upper arm to support his head and shoulders and your other hand to support his hips.

Pull the patient up on the count of three.

Pulling a Helpless Patient Up in Bed

YOU DO THIS

Follow the general rules for lifting and moving.

Pull the bed away from the wall.

Lock the wheels of the bed.

Stand behind the head of the bed.

Climb onto the leg brace of the bed or onto a small stool.

Bend over the head of the bed and reach your hands over the patient's shoulders to grasp his axillae or armpits.

Pull the patient up by straightening your back.

Using a Drawsheet to Roll and Lift

YOU DO THIS

Follow the general rules for lifting and moving.

Fold a drawsheet in quarters and lay it beneath the patient so that it is under his body from the shoulders to the thighs.

To turn the patient toward you, face the side of the bed and grasp the far edges of the drawsheet near the patient's shoulder and hip; then pull the sheet to you.

The quartered drawsheet may also be used by two people to pull a very heavy person up in the bed.

YOU DO THIS

Follow the general rules for lifting and moving.

Lifters stand on either side of the bed and face each other.

Each lifter grasps the quartered drawsheet at the patient's shoulder and hip.

On the count of three they pull the drawsheet upward.

Encouraging Your Patient to Help Himself Turn and Sit Up

A patient can turn himself by using a side rail. Have him lie on his back with knees flexed and grasp the rail with his far hand. Then he can pull himself over.

A patient can raise himself to a sitting position by pulling on a length of rope tied securely to the center of the footstead of the bed.

A patient can use an overhead trapeze to move himself when in bed.

These methods are often taught as part of training in activities of daily living. It is your duty to see that the patient performs them.

POSITIONING YOUR PATIENT IN A CHAIR

The way you position and support the geriatric patient to sit in a chair is very important. It can make the difference between his comfort and desire to sit and his fatigue, pain, and unwillingness to sit (Fig. 35).

YOU DO THIS

Keep the patient's spine straight and the body in line.

Place the lower part of the back against the back of the chair so that body weight is equally distributed between thighs and buttocks.

See that lower legs are at right angles to thighs.

Place the feet flat.

Place arms on armrests so that they are supported and help maintain body balance.

Use pillows and footstools to correct sitting alignment.

Study Figures 36 and 37 which show poor and corrected sitting positions.

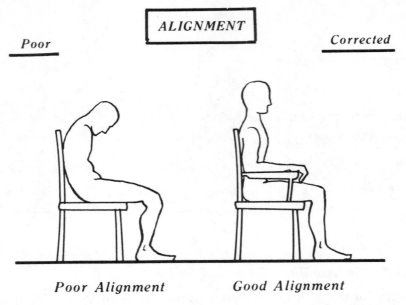

Poor   **ALIGNMENT**   Corrected

Poor Alignment   *Good Alignment*

Figure 35. Examples of good and poor positioning in a chair. (Reprinted from Elementary Rehabilitation Nursing Care, *U.S. Public Health Service, Division of Nursing.)*

Using Safety Equipment

Sometimes, for the safety of the patient, it is necessary to use a belt or chest restraint that will hold him in the chair. These should be put on so that they maintain body alignment and do not interfere with a patient's blood circulation or comfort.

USING A WHEELCHAIR

(*See* Your Geriatric Patient Needs Adaptive Equipment.)

Transferring Your Patient Into a Wheelchair

YOU DO THIS:

Place the wheelchair facing the bedside stand, with its back near the foot of the bed.

Raise the footrests.

Set the brakes on the chair or secure the chair against a wall or piece of heavy furniture.

If the bed has brakes, set them, or put stops under the rollers.

Place pressure pad in the wheelchair. If necessary, arrange a blanket.

Help the patient dress. Lower the bed level, or position a footstool for the patient's feet.

Poor   *Corrected*

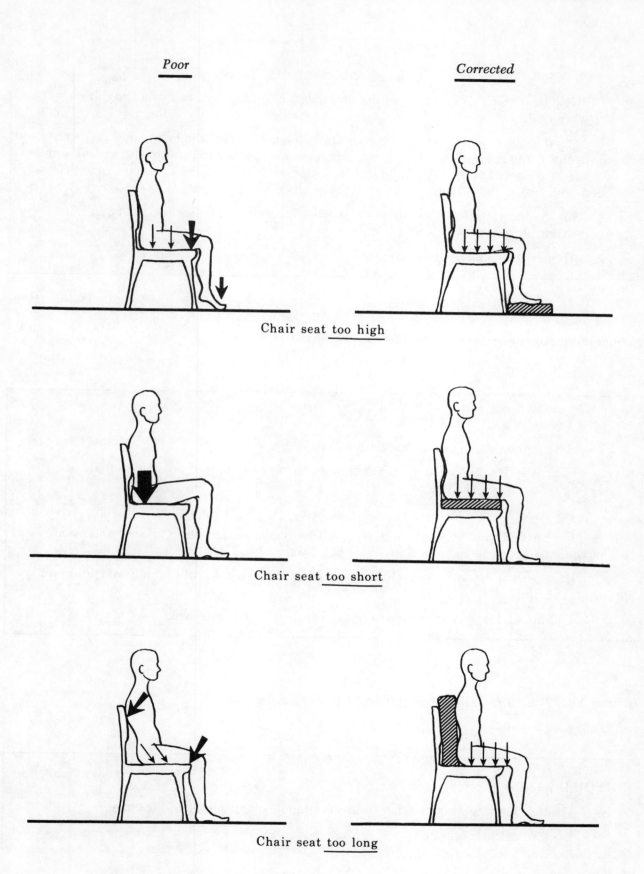

Chair seat <u>too high</u>

Chair seat <u>too short</u>

Chair seat <u>too long</u>

Figures 36 and 37. Examples of poor sitting positions that have been corrected. (Reprinted from
Elementary Rehabilitation Nursing Care, *U.S. Public Health Service, Division of Nursing.)*

163

YOUR GERIATRIC PATIENT NEEDS SLEEP, REST, POSITIONING, AND TRANSFERRING

Help the patient to a sitting position in the bed and dangle his feet over the side near the wheelchair.

Stand at the patient's side, place your arm around his waist, and help him stand, step to the floor, and get into the chair. Another method is to stand in front of the patient with your right leg between his legs. Support him with your hands under his armpits, or axillae, bend your knees, and lift and pivot him into the chair.

Put the footrests down and place the patient's feet on them. See that his body is in good sitting alignment.

Arrange the blanket around his body.

Helping Your Patient to Transfer from Bed to Wheelchair

YOU DO THIS

Have patient sit on side of bed with legs dangling.

Place wheelchair at an angle facing the bed and as close to it as possible so that patient's legs are between bed and chair.

Lock wheelchair brakes.

Have patient place his hand that is closest to the wheelchair on its armrest and place his other hand on the bed and close to his buttocks.

Have patient lift and pivot into the wheelchair, bearing most of his body weight on his hands and arms.

This method is used in reverse to transfer from wheelchair to bed.

Helping Your Patient to Transfer from Wheelchair to Straight Chair

YOU DO THIS

Position the wheelchair so that footrests straddle one front leg of the chair.

Lock wheelchair brakes.

Have patient slide forward to the edge of the wheelchair and place his nearest hand on the seat and his other hand on the armrest.

Have the patient lift and pivot himself, bearing most of his body weight on his arms.

This method is used in reverse to transfer from straight chair to wheelchair.

This method may be used to transfer to a lower bench or toilet.

See Chapter 10 for other instructions on the use of a wheelchair.

Transferring a Helpless Patient to a Wheelchair or Chair

YOU DO THIS:

Dress the patient.

See that he is wearing a belt (Fig. 38) or clothing with a strong waistband.

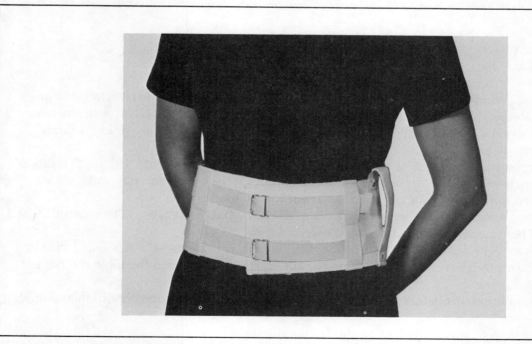

Figure 38.   A belt used in lifting a patient for transfers.   (Reprinted by permission of © J. T. Posey Co.)

Position the wheelchair.

Help the patient to sit with his legs dangling over the side of the bed.

Position his body as close to the edge as possible.

Ask the patient to relax his body and not to try to help you.

Position his arms close to his body with his hands folded in his lap.

Position his feet together and aligned under his body. Point the toes forward.

Face the patient and straddle his legs.

Position your feet so that they brace the outsides of the patient's feet.

Squeeze your legs to brace the patient's leg.

On the side toward which you will be turning, place the palm of your near hand on the patient's hip.

Grasp the center of the patient's belt or waistband with your other hand.

Then make the following movements at the same time:

> Pull on the belt or waistband.
>
> Straighten your back.
>
> Lock the patient's knee, on the side toward which you are turning, by pressing your knee against the patient's kneecap.
>
> Swivel the patient's buttocks toward and into the chair.

THE TILT TABLE

A tilt table is a special, stretcher type of table, the surface of which can be positioned at any angle from level to upright. A bed patient is moved onto and strapped to the table; then the table is tilted. Tilting is valuable to general blood circulation. It helps prevent kidney stones, urinary infection, and pressure sores.

A doctor prescribes the degree of tilt and the time period for each patient. The first elevation usually is to an angle of 20 or 30 degrees for 20 to 30 minutes. The elevation angle and time are gradually increased until the patient can remain upright for an hour.

A professional nurse should be present when a patient first uses a tilt table. The patient's blood pressure is taken before, during, and after a first use.

During each use, check the patient for pallor, dizziness, light-headedness, nausea, and sweating. Watch the feet for mottling or skin discoloration. If any of these occur, level the table and patient and notify the charge nurse.

Check the holding straps before and during use. See that they are in good condition and hold securely.

Always have help to move a patient to and from a tilt table.

YOU NEED

  tilt table

  2 or 3 tilt table straps

  pillow

  bath blanket

  2 sandbags

  overbed table

YOU DO THIS

  Dress patient in full clothing, including shoes.

  If patient has an indwelling catheter, connect it to a leg drainage bag.

  Cover the tilt table with the bath blanket.

  Position the head pillow on the table.

  Transfer the patient to the tilt table. (Use two or three people as needed.)

  Place the patient on his back in supine position.

  See that the body, head, and limbs are aligned.

  See that the feet rest against the footboard.

  Use sandbags on the outside of the feet to hold them in position.

  Fasten the tilt table straps across the knees and chest.

  Tilt the table to the prescribed angle. Note the time the procedure starts and length of time patient is to remain on table.

  Observe patient during tilting.

  Place an overbed table in front of patient so that he can support his arms, read, write, or eat if he is able to do so.

TRANSFERRING WITH A MECHANICAL LIFTER

Mechanical lifters (Fig. 39) move helpless or very fat patients with safety and ease. Lifters such as Hoyer of Porta-lift are designed to lift and hold much heavier weights than any patient. Some lifters have adjustable base widths to allow for passage through doorways. The base of a lifter should always be wide enough to prevent tipping during lifting. Lifters are operated by a hand pump. A lifter is used to transfer a patient from bed to chair or commode and from wheelchair into automobile.

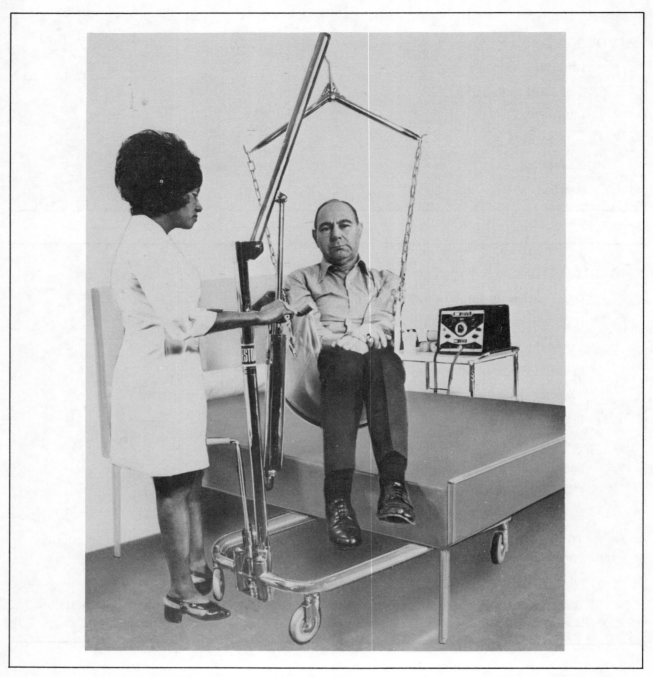

Figure 39.   A mechanical lifter used to transfer a patient from bed to chair or wheelchair, or from wheelchair to automobile. (Reprinted by permission of © J. A. Preston Corp., 1971.)

Since a patient may be fearful when using a lifter for the first time, the operation of the lifter should be explained to him and every effort made to calm his fears. Two attendants helping at that time may ease his anxiety.

Slings and harnesses should be clean, comfortable, and in safe condition.

Transferring Patient from Bed to Chair

YOU NEED

lifting machine

canvas back and seat slings. (Adjust slings to the individual, and mark adjustment points for the patient. For example, mark the particular chain link with a string.)

YOU DO THIS

Explain to the patient what you are going to do.

Place the patient on his back in supine position.

Turn the patient as necessary to position the back and seat slings. Be sure that the seat sling is under the lower part of the buttocks and above the bend of the knees.

Bring the lifter close to the bedside.

Attach the S hooks (suspended by chains from the lifter) to the back and seat slings.

Shut release knob.

Pump the handle to raise the patient above the mattress.

Check the patient and machine for good balance.

Swing the patient's feet off the bed.

Use guide handles to move the patient away from the bed.

Suspend the patient directly over the chair, commode, or other object onto which he is to be placed.

Slowly open the release knob and lower the patient onto the chair or other object.

When patient is seated, disconnect the S hooks.

Do not remove the sling supports. Leave them in place on the patient until he has been returned to bed.

Transferring Patient from Chair to Bed

Reverse the procedure.
Approach the bed with the lifter so that front wheels roll under the bed and the patient hangs directly over the bed.
Turn the patient and place his feet on the bed.
Slowly open the release valve and lower the patient into bed.
Disconnect S hooks. Remove slings by turning patient from side to side.

Special Safety Rules

If the patient is very thin or has pressure sores, protect pressure points with extra padding.

Protect the patient against skin injury from S hooks.

Always watch and protect the patient's legs and feet. Never allow them to bump against furniture or wheelchair rests.

THREE-PERSON CARRY

Rearrange furniture to allow sufficient space for turn and transfer.

Level the mattress.

Protect pressure areas with self-adhering foam.

Position the patient on his back with arms either crossed over his chest or extended along each side.

Position the stretcher or tilt table at a right angle to the foot of the bed on the side of the persons who will be lifters. The head of the stretcher should be near the bed.

Three people stand side by side and face the side of the bed from which the patient is to be lifted.

The second person counts and controls the motions.

First Person

He supports the patient's head and shoulders with one arm and places his other hand and arm under the patient's body, just below the waist. (A small pillow under the patient's head can be included in this hold.)

Second Person

He places one arm under the patient's back, crossing it beneath the arm of the first person to support the patient's chest. He places his other hand and arm under the patient to support the thighs at the hip.

Third Person

He crosses one arm over the second person's arm to reach under and support the entire buttocks. He places his other arm under both calves.

Procedure

The second person counts to three.

On the count of one, the three people secure their holds.

On the count of two, the three people bend their knees.

On the count of three, the people lift together.

On the count of four, the people step back.

On the count of five, the people turn toward the stretcher at the foot of the bed and walk toward it.

On the count of six, they deposit the patient on the stretcher.

11

YOUR GERIATRIC PATIENT NEEDS TO HAVE HIS BED MADE

STUDY GUIDE

What type of bed and mattress should a geriatric patient have?

What is a bedboard?

What bed height is the most convenient for getting in and out of bed?

If a bed is high, what should a patient use to enter or leave it?

Which geriatric patients should have side rails?

When should side rails be raised?

What extra equipment might one find on a geriatric patient's bed?

How should the bed linen of a geriatric patient be laundered?

What type of blankets should a geriatric patient use?

When is a closed bed made?

Tell how to make a closed bed.

When is an open bed prepared?

How can you change a closed bed into an open bed?

Before you start to make an occupied bed what should you do?

How can the patient help you pull up the mattress?

How do you turn a helpless patient onto his side?

When making an occupied bed, how do you remove the soiled drawsheets?

What do you do with the plastic protective sheet?

How do you remove the under sheet?

How do you put on a clean under sheet?

How do you put on a clean drawsheet?

When do you turn your patient to his other side?

How do you finish making the bottom of the bed?

How is a bed cradle used?

How is a footboard used?

BEDMAKING AND THE GERIATRIC PATIENT

The geriatric patient on any level of nursing care needs a strong, level bed and a firm mattress. If the mattress sags, a bedboard should be used. A bedboard is a length of thin pressed wood or plastic that can be placed between the bed springs and the mattress.

Most geriatric patients who can help themselves find that it is easiest to get in and out of a low bed. If a high bed is used, a patient should always have a firm, nonskid footstool to step onto when entering or leaving the bed. Electric beds that allow easy self-adjustment of head and foot heights are desirable for all geriatric patients who are capable of using them. These are also more convenient for nursing personnel because the bed level can be raised for patient care and lowered in the intervals between care.

Side rails should be part of the bed equipment for a geriatric patient. Many nursing homes require that all beds have rails and that all rails be raised at bedtime and remain raised during the night. The rail of an occupied bed should be raised during the day if the patient is confused, ill, or feeble.

Many geriatric patients require extra equipment on their beds. One may need additional pillows, an extra blanket, a footboard, or a bed cradle. Often a patient has a favorite small pillow or blanket. A patient can be very fussy about the exact arrangement of bed equipment or clothing. When possible, every effort should be made to accommodate him.

Because skin of geriatric patients is very sensitive, soft sheets and pillowcases should be used. These should never be laundered in strong detergents or bleaches and should have extra rinsing after washing. Use of a fabric softener during laundering helps remove soil and reduce roughness. Light-weight, washable blankets are recommended and should be laundered at regular intervals set by the charge nurse and at any other time when they become soiled.

Plastic and cotton drawsheets are often used on the beds of patients who are confined to bed or who may soil bed clothes because of rectal or bladder discharge. These sheets protect the mattress and allow for quick changing of the soiled area. Smaller, plastic-backed, disposable bedpads are frequently used with or instead of drawsheets.

A CLOSED BED

A closed bed is made when no patient is assigned to it.

YOU DO THIS

Remove all bedding.

Disinfect the bed.

Remake with all clean bedding, including the blanket and plastic drawsheet.

Place fresh bedding on a chair beside the bed.

Fold the bottom sheet in half lengthwise.

Lay the lengthwise fold along the center of the mattress.

Pull the sheet toward the head until the foot edge reaches just to the mattress edge.

Open the sheet.

Tuck in the top of the sheet on the side where you stand.

Make a square corner at top.

Tuck in the side of the sheet, working from top to bottom.

Lay the folded plastic sheet across the middle of the bed with the fold at center.

Open the plastic sheet.

Place the cotton drawsheet on top of the plastic sheet and in the same way.

Be sure all plastic is covered by the cotton sheet.

Tuck in both plastic and cotton drawsheets together. The use of plastic and cotton drawsheets allows these to be changed when necessary without remaking the entire bed.

Go to the other side of the bed.

Tuck in the head of the bottom sheet and make a square corner.

Tuck the bottom sheet along the side, pulling to tighten with each tuck.

Smooth the plastic and cotton drawsheets. Tuck them in together in three tight tucks: middle, top, bottom.

Return to the bedside chair.

Fold the top sheet lengthwise and lay the fold along bed center so that the top of the sheet is just to the head edge of the mattress. Open the lengthwise fold.

Lay the lengthwise folded blanket so that the top edge of the blanket is 6 inches below the top edge of the sheet. Open the blanket.

Smooth and tuck the sheet and blanket together under the foot of the mattress.

Make a square corner and tuck once.

Lay the lengthwise folded spread on the bed so that the top edge of the spread reaches to the head edge of the mattress. Open the spread.

Smooth and tuck it under at the foot.

Make a square corner but do not tuck under the last flap; the spread side hangs free.

Go to the other side.

Complete that side in the same manner.

Return to the chair side.

Put on the pillowcase and place the pillow on the bed with the open pillowcase end facing the bedside stand.

AN OPEN BED

An open bed is prepared for patients, who are allowed out of bed.

A closed bed is changed into an open bed in preparation to receive a new patient.

An open bed is made exactly as a closed bed except, that the top of the spread is cuffed under the blanket. Then the top sheet is cuffed over the spread. Then all of the top covers are fanfolded to the foot of the bed.

AN OCCUPIED BED

YOU DO THIS

Close the screen around the patient's unit.

Tell him what you are going to do.

Lower bed rests until the mattress is flat.

Remove the spread and blanket. Leave the top sheet in place. Very often a bed is made just after the patient has had a bed bath. When this is the case the bath blanket is left on the patient while the bottom of the bed is being made. Then the clean top sheet is exchanged for the bath blanket.

Have the patient help you pull up the mattress by positioning him flat on his back with knees flexed, soles against the mattress, and arms raised overhead so that he can grasp the head of the bed. Pull together on the count of three.

Ask the patient to turn on his side with his back to you. If the patient is helpless, go to the other side of the bed, turn the patient to you and raise the side rail. Then return to the chair side of the bed. The side rail permits you to move the patient safely to the edge of the bed.

Pull the cotton drawsheet, plastic sheet, and bottom sheet free from under the mattress.

Roll the cotton drawsheet tight against the patient's back.

Lift the plastic sheet over the patient's back.

Roll the bottom sheet tight against the patient's back, exposing the mattress.

Fold a clean sheet lengthwise and lay the fold on the bed as close to the patient's back and center of bed as possible.

See that the foot of the sheet reaches just to the mattress edge.

Open the sheet and roll the top half tight against the patient's back.

Tuck the head of the sheet under the mattress and make a square corner.

Tuck the side of the sheet under the mattress, working from head to foot.

Lift the plastic sheet back over the rolled under sheet and into place.

Tuck it under the mattress.

Fold a clean drawsheet in half and lay it on the plastic sheet with the fold close to the patient.

Open the drawsheet and roll the top half tight against the patient's back.

Tuck the bottom half under the mattress.

Turn the patient to you, rolling him over the linen pushed against his back. Raise the side rail if necessary.

Go to the other side of the bed.

Lower the side rail if in use.

Pull the soiled bedding free from the mattress.

Remove the soiled bottom sheet. Pull the clean sheet from under the patient and into place.

Tuck the bottom sheet under the head of the mattress.

Pull the side tight and make a square corner.

Tuck that side, working from head to foot and pulling the sheet smooth under the patient.

Pull the plastic sheet tight and tuck it.

Pull the drawsheet tight and tuck it.

Turn the patient on his back.

Return to the chair side of the bed.

Remove the pillow from under the patient's head.

Take off the soiled case and put on a clean one.

Replace the pillow under the patient's head.

Lay the clean top sheet over the soiled top sheet.

Remove the soiled sheet from under the clean top sheet.

Adjust the top sheet so that the sides hang evenly and there is enough material for a 6-inch cuff under the patient's chin.

Place the blanket over the top sheet.

Make a pleat, for foot space, in the center foot of the blanket and sheet. Tuck these together under the mattress. This prevents pressure on the patient's feet. Such pressure can cause foot drop, or a permanent damage to the foot.

Make a square corner and tuck the side once.

Put on the spread.

Tuck under the foot (no pleat).

Make a square corner, but do not tuck the side.

Cuff the top of the spread *under* the blanket top.

Cuff the top sheet *over* the spread.

Go to the other side and finish the bed in the same manner.

Leave the patient in a comfortable position.

Unscreen the bed.

USING A BED CRADLE

A bed cradle is used to protect an injured, burned, or infected part of the body from contact with the top bedding (Fig. 40). It may also be used for the comfort of a very ill patient. The cradle may be made of metal or plastic and sized to fit the part for which it is intended: arm, foot, leg, trunk.

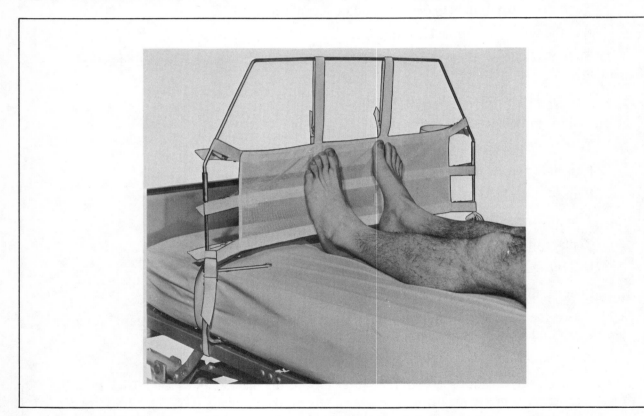

Figure 40. A bed cradle. (Reprinted by permission of © J. T. Posey Co.)

A cradle for home use can be made from a large cardboard box, available at a food market. Cut off the flaps of the open ends and one long side. Punch small holes in the other sides to allow better air circulation; then place it over the affected body part.

FOOTBOARD

A footboard is often used on the bed of an aging person who suffers from arthritis, stroke, diabetes, heart disease, kidney disease, or other condition that can cause foot trouble.

A footboard is a removable, smooth surfaced board that can be placed between the bottom edge of the mattress and the footstead of the bed (Fig. 41). It prevents top bed covers from pressing on the patient's feet. It also keeps the patient's feet in neutral position because the soles rest flat against the surface of the board. This prevents foot deformity.

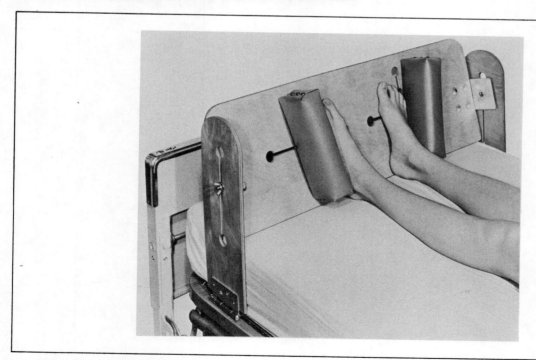

Figure 41. An adjustable footboard. (Reprinted by permission of © J. T. Posey Co.)

Footboards of various materials and several styles are available from medical supply houses. In a home situation, one can be improvised from a cardboard box, a dresser drawer, or a similar object. The best type, however, can be easily made by a local carpenter. It is made from two equal-sized pieces of 1/2-inch plywood cut 10 inches shorter than the width of the mattress. The width of the boards is the sum of 2-1/2 inches plus the length of the patients feet, plus the thickness of the mattress. The boards are joined at right angles and the angles reinforced by two 3-1/2-inch cubes of wood attached one to either side.

When put on the bed, this footboard holds very securely. One-half fits the mattress so that the mattress edge rests against the cubes. The other half fits the footstead. A special advantage to this kind of footboard is that the patient can be placed on his abdomen with his feet extending beyond the edge of the mattress and the board will hold the feet in neutral position.

12

YOUR GERIATRIC PATIENT NEEDS SKIN CARE

STUDY GUIDE

What does the skin of a geriatric patient show?

How does skin change with aging?

Do all patients receive the same skin care?

What 11 points should a skin care plan include?

What are your duties regarding diet, fluid intake, and bowel and urinary function of a patient?

What are your duties regarding the physical activity of a patient?

When should skin be inspected?

Tell ten opportunities for skin inspection.

Tell 15 places where skin should be inspected.

What do you look for during skin inspection?

What is a pressure sore or decubitus ulcer?

What are your duties regarding skin bathing and hair care of patients?

What are your duties regarding care of patients' nails and feet?

Which patients should receive back massage and oiling?

Tell how to give a back rub.

What type of bedding is useful in skin care planning for patients?

Why should bedclothing be kept clean, dry, and free of wrinkles?

What type of personal clothing should be worn?

How should bedding and personal clothing be laundered?

Why is positioning of the patient important to skin care?

What should be done when a reddened area of skin is noticed?

Tell 11 measures that can be used to relieve pressure from, and to help heal, an area of skin showing signs of pressure.

Tell how to use self-adhering foam padding.

When is a cut-out seatboard used?

Tell how to use a cut-out seatboard.

SKIN CARE IS NECESSARY

A geriatric patient's skin can reveal many things about his life. It can show his parentage, the climate in which he lived, his diet, how active he was, how long he has lived, and how filled with emotions, illnesses, and injuries his life has been. Through the years, these factors have changed his skin so that it looks different from the time of his youth.

The skin loses strength, elasticity, and ability to hold moisture and heal. It becomes folded, lined, wrinkled, lax, dry, cracked, calloused, flabby, crusty, and scarred. Dark spots, broken blood vessels, moles, and other growths appear. Head and body hair thins and grays, while ear, nose, and facial hair increases. The skin becomes less resistant to irritation, infection, injury, bruising, allergic reactions, and breakdown.

It is easy to see, then, that good skin care is a necessity for every geriatric patient. Since every patient is different, however, a skin care plan should be the one best suited to the individual patient's needs.

Any plan for good skin care of a geriatric patient must include all the following:

    a good diet
    enough fluid intake
    good bowel and urinary functions
    physical activity
    inspection of the skin
    bathing of the skin
    hair care
    care of the feet and nails
    massaging and oiling of the skin
    proper bedding and clothing
    proper body alignment

DIET, FLUID INTAKE, AND BOWEL AND URINARY FUNCTIONS

It is your duty to encourage, oversee, prepare, and help the patient in the best possible ways to eat the diet and drink the fluids that are right for him. (*See* Your Geriatric Patient Needs Food and Fluid Balance.) It is your duty to encourage, oversee, prepare, and help the patient to eliminate his body wastes in the manner best for him. (*See* Your Geriatric Patient Needs Bowel and Bladder Control.)

PHYSICAL ACTIVITY

It is your duty to encourage, oversee, prepare, and help the patient to move and change position in the best possible ways for him. This means that you must offer regular reminders to a patient that he should walk, stand, use adaptive equipment and perform activities of daily living, occupation, and recreation if he is capable of these things. To a helpless bed patient, it may mean your faithful turning of him every 2 hours. (*See* Your Geriatric Patient Needs Physical Therapy.)

INSPECTION OF THE SKIN

When to Inspect

Inspection is a very important aspect of skin care because the skin of the elderly loses sensitivity, and a patient may not feel discomfort or pain until a condition has become severe. The skin of any geriatric patient should be inspected at every opportunity.

These include:

during morning and afternoon care
during bath time
during bowel and urinary care
during dressing and undressing
before and after use of adaptive equipment
during back care
during changing of incontinent patients
during turning of bed patients
during treatments
on the complaint of any patient about itching, burning, soreness, numbness, or other changes in any part of the skin

Where to Inspect (Fig. 42)

the scalp
the hairline
behind the ears
the face and neck (especially around the mouth and eyes)
under the arms
the hands (front, back, and nails)
under the breasts
inside any large folds, or fat rolls
the elbows (front and back)
the genitals and anus
the shins and calves
the knees (front and back)
the entire back (especially the shoulder blades, spinal ridge, and buttocks)
any area that is pressured by a piece of adaptive equipment, a cast, or clothing.
any area that has been injured, bruised or shows redness or rash.

What to Look for and Report to the Charge Nurse

Texture changes: unusual smoothness, roughness, scaling, gooseflesh, graining, crusting, welts, rashes, chafing, and irritation.

Color changes: redness, blueness, graying, blackening, white spots, brown spots, and so forth.

Growths: moles, warts, tumors, callouses, corns, and so forth.

Injuries: bruises, scratches, scrapes, cuts, burns, infections, and so forth.

Pressure sores or decubitus ulcers: very red, sometimes blackened, open sores, appearing on the body where unusual pressure occurs. This can be over any bony part, such as the shoulder blades, elbows, along the spinal ridge, or heels. It can also occur under very heavy breasts or other fat rolls, and on areas rubbed by adaptive equipment or casts.

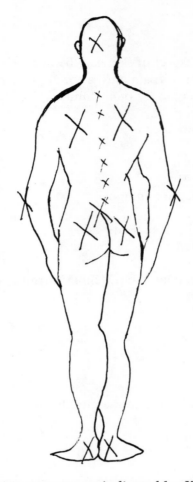

Figure 42. Body areas most subject to pressure, as indicated by Xs.

BATHING OF THE SKIN AND HAIR CARE

It is your duty to see that the patient gets the regular bathing and shampooing that is best suited to his particular needs. This may mean a weekly bath and beauty shop appointment for the active patient with very dry skin. To the incontinent patient it may mean back bathing several times a day and a bed shampoo. Special mild soaps, shampoos, and creams should be used. (*See* Your Geriatric Patient Needs to be Washed and Groomed.)

CARE OF FEET AND NAILS

It is your duty to see that fingernails and toenails of each patient receive the specific care needed by that individual. This can mean making appointments with a manicurist and a podiatrist or giving daily foot baths to a diabetic patient and arranging regular appointments with his doctor to have his nails trimmed.

MASSAGING AND OILING OF THE SKIN

Regardless of the individual bathing schedule or the level of nursing care of a geriatric patient, he should receive a back massage and oiling of body skin as part of the daily routine for morning and evening care and as often as needed.

Massage stimulates blood circulation and helps maintain skin tone. Oiling prevents drying, cracking, flaking, and crusting. Both make the patient feel and look better. Both help prevent skin from breaking down and decubitus ulcers from forming.

The face can be oiled with cleansing cream, moisturizing cream, shaving cream, or aftershave cream lotion.

Hand lotion should be used after every washing.

Special lotions, such as Lubriderm, baby lotion, and Intensive Care Lotion, are good for back care and body rubbing. These do not leave oily surfaces but soak into the skin and make it soft and pliable. Lotion should be applied at every opportunity; this means at most inspection times. Inspection and oiling the skin should be included as steps in nearly all procedures of nursing care.

Giving a Back Rub

YOU NEED

lotion (To take the chill out of the liquid, place the bottle in a pan of warm water and let stand a few minutes.)

a bath towel

YOU DO THIS

Position the patient on his far side or on his abdomen.

Expose the full back area.

Spread the towel under the patient's back and buttocks.

Apply the lotion to your hands.

Place both of your hands at the base of the spine with your fingers pointing in the direction of the neck.

Rub upward on each side of the spine, applying pressure with the palms of your hands and using long, smooth strokes to the shoulders. Then use a series of circular motions to return your hands to the base of the spine.

Repeat several times, using more lotion as needed.

Massage the buttocks with large circular movements.

Then massage in circles inside of circles until all flesh has been rubbed.

Repeat several times.

PROPER BEDDING AND CLOTHING

A firm mattress allows for better distribution of a patient's weight and therefore prevents unusual pressure on any one part of the body. It also allows for easier turning and positioning of the patient. Special mattresses that constantly redistribute body weight are available and helpful for the patient whose skin is nearing breakdown or has an existing bedsore.

Bedclothing should be kept clean, dry, and free of wrinkles. Moisture and wrinkles irritate the skin.

Soft, lightweight sheets, pillowcases, and bedcovers help prevent irritations. (*See* Your Geriatric Patient Needs to Have His Bed Made.)

Personal clothing should be loose, comfortable, soft, lightweight, and clean. Nothing that cuts off blood circulation, such as garters or elastic girdles, should be worn. Both bedclothing and personal clothing should be laundered in mild, nonirritating soap or detergent.

PROPER BODY ALIGNMENT

Positioning the patient, whether standing, sitting, or in bed, so that his weight is evenly distributed and there is no interference with blood supply is very important in maintaining skin health. (*See* Your Geriatric Patient Needs Sleep, Rest, Positioning, and Transferring.)

CARE OF A PATIENT THREATENED BY SKIN BREAKDOWN AND BEDSORES OR DECUBITUS ULCERS

Special care should be started at the first sign of redness or breakdown of the skin. The area should be inspected by the charge nurse and brought to the attention of the doctor. Measures should be taken to stop the pressure on the immediate area and to encourage healing. These procedures vary from one nursing home or doctor to another, but they may include the following:

Increased physical activity and repositioning to relieve pressure on sensitive area.

Use of a special mattress to redistribute weight constantly.

Use of a sheepskin under the back to cushion and redistribute weight and increase blood supply to the area (Fig. 43). The sheepskin is placed so that the wool is next to the patient's skin. The sheepskin may be real or synthetic. It is soft, easily washed and dried, and generally well-tolerated by the patient.

Use of self-adhering foam padding on pressure points. (Rubber rings or doughnuts are not recommended because they tend to cause other pressure points.)

Use of heel protectors (Fig. 44).

Use of normal saline solution to wash an ulcer.

Use of medication for the area (on doctor's orders).

Use of a hair dryer set on cool or of other means to dry and stimulate blood circulation to an ulcer (on doctor's orders).

Increased massaging and oiling of the surrounding area.

For an incontinent patient, a urinary catheter or condom drainage (on doctor's orders).

Use of a cut-out seatboard for a wheelchair patient (on doctor's orders).

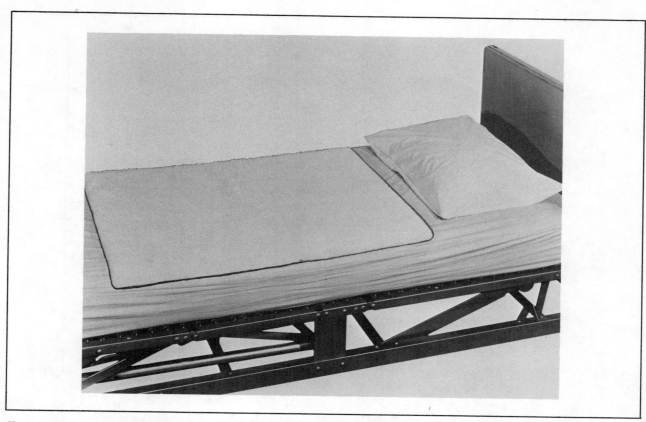

Figure 43. A synthetic sheepskin to prevent pressure sores. (Reprinted by permission of © J. T. Posey Co.)

Using Self-Adhering Foam Padding

YOU NEED

    basin with warm water

    disposable cloth or gauze sponges

    hair dryer or other blower set on cool

    foam padding

    scissors

YOU DO THIS

Clean the skin surrounding the area.

Use hair dryer set on cool to blow it dry.

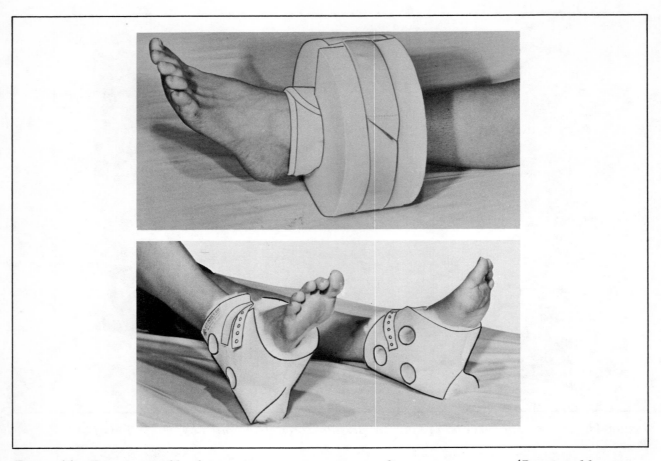

Figure 44. Two types of heel protectors to prevent or to relieve pressure sores. (Reprinted by permission of © J. T. Posey Co.)

Cut out a piece of padding three or four times larger than the sore area.

Cut a hole in the padding to the size and shape of the sore area.

Remove the adhesive liner from the pad and put the pad over the area so that the sore part is framed by the padding.

Stick the padding to the skin.

If the patient is very heavy, several pads can be stacked to make a thicker covering around the area.

Using a Cut-out Seatboard

A cut-out seatboard is ordered by the doctor to reduce pressure on the bony base of the spine when a patient uses a wheelchair. Each board is custom made for the individual patient and should never be used for another. The patient's name should be printed on the board. The board should fit the sides of the chair so that the board cannot move sideways. The board should always be used with a foam cushion, 3 or 4 inches thick.

YOU NEED

the patient's wheelchair

the patient's cut-out board

foam cushion that fits the chair seat

a pillowcase

YOU DO THIS

Inspect the seatboard for splintering edges or cracks. Report any to the charge nurse.

Place the seatboard in the wheelchair before transferring the patient.

Position the board so that the cut-out part is toward the back of the chair.

Put the pillowcase on the cushion.

Put the cushion on the seatboard.

Transfer the patient.

13

YOUR GERIATRIC PATIENT NEEDS TO BE WASHED AND GROOMED

STUDY GUIDE

Morning Care

Why should you take time and be patient with an older person on his awakening?

How should you greet a geriatric patient who has just awakened?

What four kinds of help may patients need in order to urinate?

What five kinds of help may patients need for oral hygiene?

In what six ways may patients need help with washing their faces and hands?

In what five ways may a patient need help combing his hair?

What types of help may a patient need when putting on his clothes?

What clothing should a patient put on in the morning?

Tell what you need to wash a patient's face and hands.

Tell how to wash a patient's face and hands.

Tell what you need to give oral hygiene to a patient with dentures.

Tell how to give oral hygiene to a patient with dentures.

Tell how to clean a patient's own teeth.

How do you use an electric toothbrush?

Tell how to give mouth care to a helpless patient.

Baths

What factors determine the bathing routine for a geriatric patient?

How often should a geriatric patient bathe?

At what time of day should a geriatric patient bathe?

What parts of the body should be washed daily or more often?

Give 16 general rules for giving showers and baths to geriatric patients.

Why is a shower often preferred to a bath for a geriatric patient?

Tell what you need to help give a shower?

Tell how to give a shower.

Tell what you need to help give a tub bath.

Tell what you do before giving a tub bath.

Tell what you do during the bath.

Tell what you do after the bath.

What do you need to give a sitz bath?

How do you give a sitz bath?

Tell what you need to give a foot bath.

How do you give a foot bath?

Tell what you need to give a bed bath.

Tell how to give a bed bath.

Tell how to give a partial bed bath.

What should you do after a bed bath?

Nail Care

What do you need in order to give nail care?

Tell how to give nail care.

Shaving

What do you need in order to shave a patient?

Tell how to shave a patient.

Hair Care

What is the preferred means of giving hair care to geriatric patients?

What should you do when a patient has self-care equipment for giving hair care?

Give the general rules for shampooing a geriatric patient's hair.

Where is the best place to give a shampoo?

Tell what you need and how to give a shampoo at a sink.

Tell what you need and how to give a shampoo in bed.

Tell what you need and how to comb a patient's hair.

Evening Care

What do you need in order to give evening care?

How do you give evening care?

MORNING CARE

On awakening, most people feel the need to urinate, clean their mouths, wash their faces and hands, comb their hair, and dress before breakfast. Your geriatric patients have these wants, too, but they may require more time and more help to accomplish them than does the average adult patient.

The Geriatric Patient on Awakening

Old people are often stiff when they awaken, and movement may be slow and painful. Time must be allowed for this, and your patience is necessary. Geriatric patients dislike being rushed, and if pushed, may resist instead of cooperating.

Old people are sometimes confused on awakening and need to be oriented. The way that you greet them can mean the difference between relative independence and total dependence.

Your greeting should establish in the patient's mind who he is, who you are, where you are, what time it is, what you are going to do, and what is expected of him. Speak in a cheerful voice that is clear and distinct. Speak in short sentences.

You may need to repeat the information. Often the patient will question you.

Example:

You: Good Morning, Mr. Brown. It's Miss Jones, your aide. Time to get up. Breakfast is almost ready. You know how you enjoy breakfast at Cadbury House.
Patient: Who did you say you are?
You: I'm Miss Jones. I help you to get ready for breakfast.
Patient: Oh — oh — yes. Is it breakfast time?
You: Yes, it is, Mr. Brown. Eight o'clock is breakfast time at Cadbury House.
Patient: Cadbury House? I must have been dreaming. I thought I was home with my wife.
You: No, Mr. Brown. You're here at Cadbury House with your friends. Now, let me help you to get out of bed so you can go to the bathroom.
Patient: All right, Miss _____?
You: Miss Jones. I help you every morning. I'm going to put the bed rail down so that you can get up for breakfast.
Patient: Oh sure — Miss Jones — I didn't quite — I didn't quite recognize you, Miss Jones.
You: Do you want me to help you with your slippers, Mr. Brown?
Patient: That's all right. I can do it myself.
You: I put the light on in the bathroom for you. The clothes that you wanted are there on your chair. After you get dressed, I'll help you along the hall to the dining room.
Patient: What are we having for breakfast today?

You can see by this example that the orienting process can be slow and require your attention, but it gets the day off to a good start for your patient. (*See* Your Geriatric Patient Needs Remotivation and Resocialization.)

Levels of Morning Care

Morning care for some patients may be no more than what is indicated in the preceding example. Others may need much more help.
To urinate, a patient may require one of the following:
      help in walking to the bathroom
      help in using a commode
      a bedpan or urinal
      care for incontinence

To give oral hygiene, a patient may require one of the following:

    a reminder to brush his teeth

    preparation of mouthwash and toothbrush

    preparation of activities of daily living (A.D.L.) equipment for tooth care

    your brushing of his teeth

    special mouth care for a very ill or unconscious patient

To wash his face and hands a patient may require:

    a reminder to do so in the bathroom

    preparation of water and washcloth in the bathroom

    preparation of A.D.L. aids

    a basin of water and washcloth, soap, and towel at bedside

    your washing of his face

    a prepackaged, disposable washcloth if he is in bed

To comb his hair, the patient may require:

    a reminder to do so

    preparation of comb, mirror, and other equipment

    preparation of A.D.L. equipment

    partial help with combing

    complete combing by you

To dress, the patient may require:

    no help

    a reminder to do so

    some help

    preparation of A.D.L. aids

    total help

Which clothing a patient puts on in the morning is determined by a number of factors:

    the level of nursing care that he is receiving

    where he is going to eat his breakfast

    the regulations of the nursing facility

    the patient's wishes

Many nursing homes require that independent residents assigned to the main dining room wear street clothes to all meals. Others allow robes and slippers at breakfast.

Patients who require constant medical supervision usually have their meals in a small dining room on the same floor as the care unit. The treatment schedule of these patients often determines whether they dress in robes or street clothes for breakfast. Some may have breakfast in their rooms.

Patients on an acute care unit are usually confined to bed and are served all meals at bedside or sometimes at chairside in the room.

Patients in a long-term care unit for chronic brain syndrome are usually dressed in hospital gowns and washable robes for breakfast.

Washing the Patient's Face and Hands

YOU NEED

    basin of warm water (100°F)

    washcloth

face towel

soap in a dish

YOU DO THIS

Position him and place the equipment so that he can wash himself. If the patient cannot wash himself, you bathe him.

Dip the cloth in the clear water.

Wring it well and make a mitt to cover your hand.

Wipe the patient's eyes, starting at the nose and wiping outward.

Then wipe the rest of the face.

Do not use soap on the face unless the patient wants it.

Put the towel on the bed by the patient's near hand.

Put the basin on the towel.

Place both of the patient's hands in the basin.

Do not put the cake of soap into the water.

Soap your own hands and use them to soap the patient's.

Use the washcloth to rinse the hands.

Remove the basin.

Wipe the patient's hands on the towel.

Oral Hygiene, or Mouth Care

Dentures, or False Teeth

YOU NEED

toothbrush

solution of dentifrice for artificial dentures, such as Kleenite or Polident

gauze square or tissue

YOU DO THIS

Clean dentures before giving other mouth care.

Remove a full denture by grasping it with a piece of gauze or tissue and tilting it away from the gums.

Remove a partial denture by lifting the metal clamp with your fingernail.

Soak dentures in the solution of dentifrice.

Take the dentures to the bathroom or utility room. Hold one denture at a time, in the palm of your hand, over a sink partly filled with water and brush under running water.

Place the dentures in a clean cup of clean water.

Return to the patient and place the dentures in a safe place.

Clean the patient's own teeth and allow him to rinse his mouth with mouthwash.

The Patient's Own Teeth

YOU NEED

toothbrush

toothpaste

a glass of mouthwash or water

emesis basin

a face towel

tissues

a drinking straw, if desired

YOU DO THIS

Follow the general rules for treatments.

Spread the face towel under the patient's chin.

Hold the toothbrush over the emesis basin and pour mouthwash or water onto the brush.

Apply a small amount of toothpaste to the brush.

If the patient is able to brush his teeth, hand him the brush.

Hold the emesis basin under the patient's chin.

If he is unable to brush his teeth, you insert the brush into his mouth and gently brush, using up and down strokes.

Let the patient rinse his mouth and spit into the emesis basin.

Wipe his mouth with a tissue and then with the towel.

Electric Toothbrush

This type of toothbrush may be used by the patient with limited range of motion or muscle weakness. Both plug-in and battery-operated toothbrushes are used in much the same way as an ordinary toothbrush. Apply the toothpaste before turning on the toothbrush. Before helping a patient to use an electric toothbrush, be sure that you know the correct way to operate it.

Special Mouth Care for the Helpless Patient

YOU NEED

tongue depressor wrapped with gauze bandage

cup of mouthwash solution

emesis basin

towel

YOU DO THIS

Turn the patient's head to one side.

Spread the towel beneath his chin.

Dip the wrapped tongue depressor in mouthwash solution until it is wet but not dripping. Take the patient's cheeks on both sides of the mouth between the thumb and fingers of one hand. Squeeze gently to open the patient's mouth. Insert the depressor between the patient's lips.

Swab the teeth, gums, and tongue with the depressor.

Repeat as often as necessary to clean.

Change the gauze on the tongue depressor if necessary.

This mouth care should be given every hour or so to unconscious or otherwise helpless patients. A thin application of oil to the lips helps prevent cracking.

A coated tongue and foul breath are often part of illnesses that cause unconsciousness or helplessness. Also, the mouth of an unconscious or helpless patient tends to drop open and this causes the mouth to dry. Frequent mouth care relieves these conditions and adds to a patient's comfort.

BATHS

Several factors determine the bathing routine for a geriatric patient:
> his doctors orders
> his overall physical condition
> his day-to-day physical condition
> his need for a bath
> the routine of a nursing home
> his wishes about bathing

How Often

Many geriatricians think that a daily tub bath or shower is not good for a patient. It is their opinion that daily bathing is too tiring and too drying for the skin, and exposes the patient to unnecessary chilling and falling. They think that once or twice a week is often enough for the geriatric patient to bathe. Other doctors claim that any bad effects of daily bathing are less than the desirable effects of the general activity, blood stimulation, and sense of well-being produced by being clean and cared for.

The patient who is active and physically fit is better able to tolerate frequent bathing than is one with a condition that causes unusual pain.

The patient with a short-term illness, such as a cold, may need to discontinue tub or shower bathing during the illness.

The patient who is incontinent certainly needs a bath more frequently than a patient who has good body control.

Bath routines in nursing facilities differ according to the thinking of the doctors on the staff, the nursing director, the level of care given by the facility (such as self-care or chronic brain syndrome), and the number of nursing personnel available to give care.

The patient's wishes also play a large part in the plan for his care. It is cruel to needlessly deny this pleasure to a person who throughout his lifetime enjoyed a daily bath. It is equally cruel to insist that a person must bathe whether or not he needs or likes it.

What Time of Day

The time for a bath should also be flexible. Some patients like to bathe in the evening. Others in the afternoon or as soon as they awaken in the morning. Whenever possible, allowances should be made for such preferences.

Daily Care

Regardless of how often a full bath is given to a patient, certain parts of the body should get washing and other skin care daily or several times daily.

MEETING YOUR GERIATRIC PATIENT'S NEEDS

These are:
    face
    hands
    underarms
    genitals
    feet
    bony parts (elbows, knees, spine)
(*See* Your Geriatric Patient Needs Skin Care and Your Geriatric Patient Needs Bowel and Bladder Control.)

When giving any kind of bath to a patient, the safety of the patient must be a prime consideration. Special safety equipment and rules are discussed in another part of this book. (*See* Your Geriatric Patient Needs a Clean Safe Comfortable Place).

General Rules for Giving Showers and Baths

See that the bathroom is clean, warm, and draft-free.

Help lay out the patient's clean clothes in his room.

See that the patient's room is warm and draft-free.

See that special equipment (eyeglasses, hearing aids) are safely stored.

See that the patient has with him any necessary adaptive equipment (soap on string, long-handled brush).

Take the patient to the bathroom in a wheelchair if possible.

If a shower bench or regular chair is to be used, place it in the shower stall before the patient enters.

Turn on and test the strength, direction, and temperature of the shower spray *before the patient enters.* Adjust the spray to a gentle one, aimed to reach the patient below shoulder level. The temperature should be warm (100°F.) — never hot. Fill the tub and test the water temperature (100°F.) before the patient enters.

Unless a shampoo is intended, see that the patient wears a shower cap.

Remove a condom urinary drainage set if the patient is wearing one.

Be sure brakes are locked on a shower chair while it is in the stall.

Even when the patient is able to bathe himself, do not leave him alone in the bathroom.

Help the patient to wash himself, as needed, but allow him to do as much as possible for himself.

Do not allow the patient to stay longer than necessary in the shower or bath.

Do not expose the patient unnecessarily.

Wear a plastic apron to protect yourself.

Shower

For the geriatric patient, a shower is often the preferred means of bathing. It is easier and safer than transferring in and out of a tub. It takes less time and causes less strain on a patient. A shower chair can be rolled into the shower and allows the patient greater security and comfort.

A shower chair is a small sized straight chair on wheels. On some, the chair seat is cut out for easier bathing of the genitals. Some types can be used as bath, commode, and shower chairs (Fig. 45). Wheels on the chair can be locked.

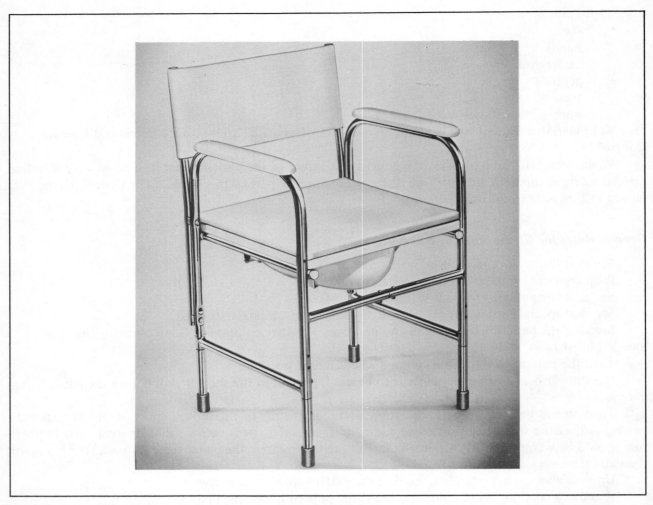

Figure 45.   A combination commode and shower chair. (Reprinted by permission of © J. A. Preston Corp., 1971.)

Helping Give a Shower

YOU NEED

     soap

     A.D.L. bath aids

     shower cap or shampoo

     1 or 2 towels

     washcloth

     shower chair, bench, or standard, strong, straight chair

terry robe or bath blanket

skin lotion

deodorant

large plastic apron

YOU DO THIS

Follow general rules for showers.

Take patient to shower area.

Put on the plastic apron.

If a bench or standard chair is used in the stall, fold one towel and lay it on the seat; this is not necessary with a shower chair.

See that shower cap if needed is on patient.

Turn on water and adjust it.

If a bench or standard chair is used, help the patient to transfer to it; if a shower chair is used, help the patient to transfer to it, wheel it into the shower stall, and lock the brakes.

See that the patient has at hand and uses A.D.L. bath aids, as needed.

Help the patient to wash and rinse if necessary.

Check the patient's genitals and buttocks. Be sure they are clean. If rash or redness is present, report it to the charge nurse.

When patient is clean, turn off shower.

Help patient to leave the shower stall.

Remove shower cap.

Help patient to dry himself thoroughly.

Apply skin lotion and observe skin condition. (Report any abnormal conditions to charge nurse.)

Wrap patient in terry robe or bath blanket.

Take patient's A.D.L. bath aids.

Leave shower room neat and clean.

Return patient to his room and help him to dress, as needed.

Tub Bath

Many nursing homes use special mechanical lifts installed next to bathtubs, to lift and deposit a patient into the tub and to remove the patient from the tub (Fig. 46). These are useful for patients with problems of balance. Before using such a lift, be sure that you learn to operate it correctly.

199

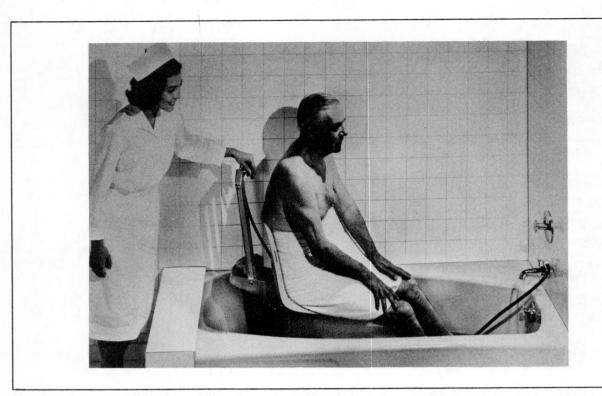

Figure 46. A mechanical lifter for the bathtub. (Reprinted by permission of © J. A. Preston Corp., 1971.)

Helping Give a Tub Bath

YOU NEED

bath towel

bath blanket or large towel

1 cloth bath mat

2 rubber suction mats

2 washcloths

soap

bath thermometer

a stool the same height as the tub

a straight chair the same height as the tub

deodorant

skin lotion

MEETING YOUR GERIATRIC PATIENT'S NEEDS

powder

clean clothing

comb and brush

YOU DO THIS

Before Bath

Drape the bath blanket over the straight chair and set it aside.

Put one rubber mat in the tub and one rubber mat on the floor beside the tub.

Cover the floor mat with the cloth mat.

Fill the tub one-third full with water at 100°F.

Have washcloth and soap at hand.

Place the stool next to the tub at a spot about one-third the tub length from the tub back, so that the patient will have access to the tub handrails.

Bring the patient to the bath area in a wheelchair. Lock the wheels of the chair and transfer the patient to the stool.

Help the patient to undress.

During Bath

Help the patient to lift one leg at a time over the edge of the tub and into the water.

Instruct the patient to take hold of the near handrail to steady himself (Fig. 47).

Stand in back of the patient and help him to ease into the tub.

Instruct him to grasp the far handrail as soon as he is able.

Help lower the patient into the tub until he is sitting comfortably.

Help the patient to bathe. (Give him one washcloth; you use the other.)

Be sure genitals are cleaned well.

Unless the patient is spastic (has uncontrollable body movements), drain the tub before helping him out of it.

Remove the bath stool and put the chair draped with the bath blanket next to the tub.

Instruct the patient to take hold of both safety hand rails.

Stand in front of the patient and help him to lift himself onto the tub edge.

Put the bath towel over his shoulders.

Help the patient to lift one leg over the side of the tub.

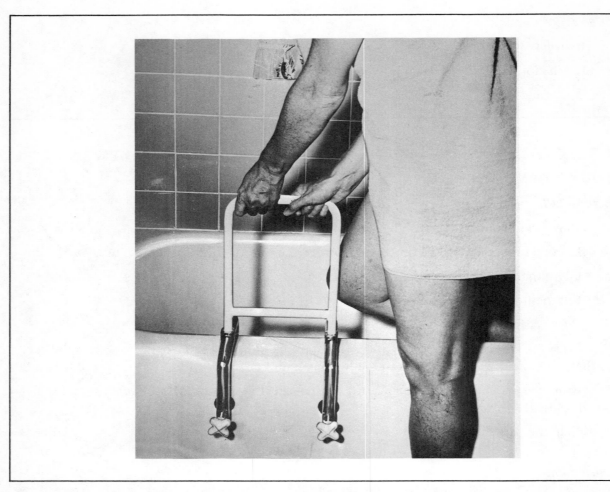

Figure 47. A hand rail for the bathtub. (Reprinted by permission of © J. A. Preston Corp., 1971.)

Help the patient to stand and move onto the straight chair.

Help the patient to remove his other leg from the tub.

Wrap the bath blanket around the patient to dry him.

Remove the towel from the patient's shoulders, and use it to dry him thoroughly.

Apply skin lotion to all of the patient's body.

Apply deodorant and bath powder.

After Bath

Help patient to dress in clean clothing.

Help him into wheelchair.

Return him to his room.

Scrub bath tub and rubber mats.

Hang mats to dry.

Put away patient's clothing.

Be sure bathroom floor is left clean and dry.

Face, hands, underarms, and genitals may be washed by the able patient in the bathroom or at bedside. Help the patient only as needed, and see that he uses A.D.L. aids, if ordered.

Sitz Bath

A sitz bath allows a patient to soak his buttocks and genitals without wetting the rest of his body (Fig. 48).

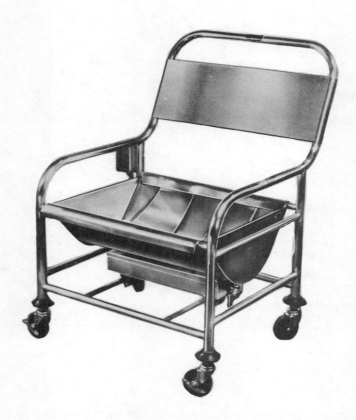

Figure 48.   A portable sitz bath. (Reprinted by permission of © J. A. Preston Corp., 1971.)

YOU NEED

a strong, straight, low chair

a plastic sheet

2 towels

1 washcloth

1 small basin large enough for the patient's buttocks

enough water at 100°F. to fill the basin one-third full

soap

skin lotion and powder

YOU DO THIS

Drape plastic sheet over chair seat.

Cover plastic sheet with folded towel.

Fill basin one-third full with water.

Place basin on chair.

Help patient remove lower clothing. (Socks and stockings may be left on. Roll stockings below knees.)

Help patient to sit in basin.

Help patient to wash himself, if necessary.

Help patient to stand and dry himself.

Inspect genitals and buttocks for redness or irritation.

Help patient to apply lotion and powder.

Help patient to get dressed.

Remove and clean equipment.

Genital Bath or Perineal Care

The patient with common geriatric problems such as urinary dribbling or rectal leaking requires frequent daily genital and rectal washing. Here is a simple and quick way for either the patient or you to bathe his genital and rectal area.

YOU NEED

    1 large pitcher of warm (100°F) soapy water

    1 large pitcher of warm (100°F) clear water

    2 disposable washcloths

    plastic disposal bag

    skin lotion

    clean genital pad or dressing

YOU DO THIS

    Remove soiled genital pad. Put it in plastic disposal bag.

    Seat the patient on the toilet, commode, or bedpan.

    Pour the soapy water slowly over the genital and rectal area.

    Use one washcloth to clean off soil. Wipe in one direction only — from front to back.

    Discard washcloth into disposal bag.

    Pour clear water over the genital and rectal area.

    Pat dry with second washcloth. Dry from front to back.

    Discard washcloth into disposal bag.

    Help patient off the toilet, commode, or bedpan.

    Apply skin lotion

    Put on clean genital pad or dressing.

Foot Bath

A foot bath allows a patient to soak and clean his feet without wetting the rest of his body.

YOU NEED

    a comfortable chair

    a plastic sheet

    a bath mat or towel

a towel

a washcloth

a basin large enough to hold the patient's feet

enough water at 100°F, to fill the basin one-third full

soap

skin lotion and powder

YOU DO THIS

Help the patient to remove his shoes and stockings or socks. See that his pants are rolled up or removed.

Place plastic sheet under patient's feet.

Place bath mat over plastic sheet.

Fill basin one-third full and place on mat near patient's feet.

Help patient to place his feet in water.

Help patient, as needed, to wash feet.

Remove feet from basin.

Help to dry thoroughly.

Inspect condition of feet. (Report unusual findings.)

Give nail care if needed.

Apply lotion and powder.

Help patient to get dressed.

Clean and put away equipment.

A Complete Bed Bath

YOU NEED

1 bath towel

1 face towel

1 washcloth

bath blanket

clean bed linen (if the bed is to be made)

comb and brush

hair tonic or cream

soap in a dish

skin lotion

alcohol or skin lotion and bath powder. (The choice of alcohol or lotion would depend on the patient's skin. Alcohol would be used on oily skin, lotion on dry.)

large basin of water at 100°F temperature. Test it with a bath thermometer. This is the ideal temperature to prevent chilling or burning the patient. Bring the water last so that it won't cool through waiting.

nailbrush, scissors, file or emery board, hand lotion

YOU DO THIS

Lower the bed if elevated and if lowering is allowed

Remove unneeded pillows. One can be left under the head if the patient desires.

Put on the bath blanket as you fanfold the top covers to the foot of the bed. Be sure the feet are free.

Face, Neck, and Ears

Remove the patient's gown.

Lift the patient's head and spread the large towel across his pillow.

Spread the face towel under his chin.

Wet the washcloth and wring it so it does not drip.

Make a bath mitt of the cloth by wrapping it around your palm and fingers, holding it with the thumb. Tuck the edges under so they don't drag.

Wash the eyes gently, from the nose outward, with plain water. Use a separate corner of the washcloth for each eye.

Wash the face, forehead, nose, and cheeks with plain water. (Use soap only if necessary.)

Rinse in the same way.

Do not put the soap into the bath water at any time.

Wrap a corner of the face towel around your hand to prevent its dragging, and dry the face.

Wash the neck and ears in the same way. Wash the far ear first, then the neck, then the near ear.

Rinse and dry.

Chest and Abdomen

Remove the towel from under the patient's head and spread it across the chest.

Pull the bath blanket and other towel down to the abdomen.

Soap, rinse, dry, and observe the chest and sides of the chest, working under the towel. Pay special attention to the area under the breasts.

Apply skin lotion to the chest and under breasts.

Leave the towel over the chest. Pull the bath blanket lower to expose the entire abdomen.

Soap, rinse, dry, and observe the abdomen, sides of abdomen, the upper part of the hips, and the front pubic area. Use long, smooth strokes to avoid pressure and tickling.

Apply skin lotion.

Pull up the blanket and remove the towels.

Arms and Hands

Bring the far arm and shoulder across the patient's chest.

Place the large towel under the arm.

Soap, rinse, dry, and observe the arm, including the axilla (or armpit).

Apply skin lotion

Remove the towel and place it under the near arm.

Soap, rinse, and dry the arm, including the axilla.

Apply skin lotion.

Remove the towel and spread it on the bed under the patient's near hand.

Put the basin on the towel and have the patient put both hands into the water.

Soap your hands and use them to soap the patient's hands. Use a nailbrush, if needed.

Rinse. Remove the basin. Dry the hands thoroughly. Apply skin lotion. Observe the hands and give nail care as needed.

Legs and the Feet

Arrange the bath blanket to expose the far leg and cover the rest of the body.

Have the patient flex (bend) the far knee.

Spread the towel under the leg.

MEETING YOUR GERIATRIC PATIENT'S NEEDS

Soap, rinse, dry, and observe the leg.

Apply skin lotion.

Repeat the procedure with the near leg.

Flex both knees.

Place the towel on the bed between the feet. Place the basin on the towel.

Lift the feet into the basin and allow them to soak. If the feet are large or the patient helpless, bathe one foot at a time in the basin.

Soap with your hands. Use the nailbrush, if needed. Rinse. Remove the basin and place the feet on the towel.

Dry well between the toes. Observe and give nail care as needed.

Apply lotion. Remove towel.

Back and Buttocks (or Hips)

Help the patient turn onto his far side or onto his abdomen. Adjust his position so that he is comfortable and you can work comfortably.

Change the bath water.

Uncover the patient's back.

Spread the large towel under his back and buttocks.

Soap, rinse, dry, and observe the patient's neck, back, and buttocks. Use long, firm strokes.

Rub the patient's back, giving special attention to pressure areas (shoulders and hips). Apply skin lotion. (See "Giving a Back Rub" in preceding chapter.)

Return the patient onto his back.

Genitalia

Put a towel under the patient's buttocks.

Place the bath basin, soap, and towel within the patient's reach and, if he is able, allow him to wash, rinse, and dry himself.

If he is unable, you must do it for him.

It is easiest to wash a patient's genitals by placing him on a bedpan. Then use a pitcher to pour some warm water over the genitals. Use the cloth mitt to soap the genitals. Pour more water to rinse. Dry well. The towel and cloth used to bathe genitals should not be reused until laundered.

YOU NEED

the same equipment as for a bed bath

YOU DO THIS

Position the patient comfortably.

Place all the equipment within his reach.

Allow him to bathe all of himself but his back and feet.

Wash his feet in the same way as for a bed bath.

Allow him to wash his genitals.

Apply skin lotion to entire body.

After a Bath

Give mouth care. (This may be done before the bath if desired.)

Spread a towel under the patient's head.

Help him to comb and arrange his hair.

Allow the patient to use deodorant, cologne, or makeup, if desired.

Help the patient into a clean gown.

Make the bed with clean linen.

Clean and put away equipment.

Report any unusual condition observed during the bath.

NAIL CARE

When the services of a beauty parlor are available, many male and female patients choose to have their fingernails cared for by a beautician. The services of a podiatrist are usually available for older people, and this insures good foot care. (Medicare pays for such services.) If these services are unavailable, however, you should give total nail care. You should always observe the nails at bath time and correct immediate problems, such as broken nails or hangnails. A doctor or podiatrist should cut the toenails of a diabetic patient.

YOU NEED

    plastic sheet

    small wash basin half filled with water at 100°F.

    soap

    orangewood stick

    skin lotion

    soft nailbrush

    nail scissors or clippers

    emery board

YOU DO THIS

    Position the patient comfortably near a table.

    Cover tabletop with plastic.

    Fold towel and put over plastic.

    Bring basin with water.

    Help patient to place hands in water.

    Allow patient's hands to soak and wash.

    Clean the nails well, using orange stick and nailbrush.

    Bring clean water to rinse hands and nails.

    Dry hands and nails thoroughly.

    Trim nails with clippers or scissors. Cut straight across, not around the nail.

    Remove rough edges with emery board.

    Apply skin lotion.

SHAVING A MALE PATIENT

YOU NEED

    a tray with: razor and blades

                  paper towels

bowl of warm water

shaving cream or soap

2 towels

basin of hot water

after-shave lotion

YOU DO THIS

Have a good light on the patient's face.

Have the patient sit erect, if allowed.

Spread one towel under his chin.

Dip other towel in the basin of hot water.

Wring it as dry as possible.

Place it over the lower face and chin for several minutes. This softens the whiskers.

Put some shaving cream in the palms of your hands and rub your palms over the patient's face. This way you control the area covered with cream.

Use a paper towel to wipe your hands.

Stretch the patient's skin tight at all times. This prevents cutting the skin.

To shave, stroke upward in a long, smooth movement. Follow it with a similar stroke downward over the same area. This makes a close, neat shave, since all hairs do not grow in the same direction.

Position the patient's head as needed to help you.

Clean the razor on paper towels to remove hairs.

Dip the razor in the bowl of warm water to remove hairs.

Run steaming water over the face towel.

Wring it as dry as possible and spread over the shaved area for several minutes.

Pat the face dry with the neck towel.

Apply shaving lotion to the palms of your hands and massage over the shaved area.

If you should cut the skin, use a styptic pencil to touch the spot. This stops the bleeding.

HAIR CARE

A geriatric patient needs regular hair care: combing, washing, cutting, and setting. Groomed hair is not only necessary for personal cleanliness but it also gives a person a sense of well-being and is attractive to others. Because of these facts, many nursing facilities have beauty parlors and barber shops or arrange for their services to be brought to the patients on a regular basis. Whenever possible, this is the preferred means of washing, cutting, and setting hair.

Not all patients can afford these services or are able to make use of them. When this is so, the charge nurse must see that patients receive hair care. You should tell the charge nurse if a patient seems in need of a shampoo or a haircut. She must approve every shampoo and haircutting. Sometimes a doctor's order may be necessary for a shampoo and a signed permission required for a haircut. The hair of geriatric patients tends to be dry. A mild shampoo should be used and if indicated, a cream rinse.

It is understood, however, that you supervise the daily grooming needs of your patients. You see that the patient's hair is combed and neat, you help female patients use hairsetting equipment, and you see that patients use any self-care equipment for this purpose.

Two types of hairsetting equipment are very useful to patients with limited use of hands or arms. They are Velcro self-fastening rollers and hair tape. The latter is very comfortable for use in bed.

When the charge nurse does tell you to shampoo a patient's hair, several choices are possible, and she will select the one that is most convenient and comfortable for the patient.

They are:

shampoo in shower
shampoo at sink
shampoo in bed

General Rules for Shampooing

See that the room is warm and draft-free.
Don't expose the patient's body more than necessary.
Protect the patient's clothing.
Handle the patient as gently as possible.
Brush hair before shampooing to help loosen dirt from scalp.
See that the patient's eyes are protected.
Plug ears with cotton to prevent water from running into them.
Test water temperature before using. It should be no hotter than 105°F.
Use as little shampoo as possible.
Massage head with fingertips — never with nails.
A shampoo in the shower is best for any patient who can tolerate it.

Giving a Shampoo at a Sink

YOU NEED

portable shower hose

plastic sheet

small sponge pad

2 towels

shampoo

washcloth

cotton earplugs

hairbrush

portable electric dryer

YOU DO THIS

Place patient in wheelchair or straight chair, positioned close to and facing sink.

Put plastic sheet around patient's neck and shoulders.

Put towel over plastic sheet.

Brush patient's hair.

Attach shower hose; turn on and test water.

Lean patient forward in chair so that head is over sink.

Put sponge pad under patient's chin.

Put earplugs in patient's ears.

Give patient washcloth to hold over eyes.

Wet hair, apply shampoo, and massage scalp.

Rinse.

Apply shampoo again and rinse.

Turn off water.

Wring hair gently.

Sit patient upright, and remove eye pad and earplugs.

Bring shoulder towel around head. Dry hair.

Remove plastic sheet.

Replace with dry towel.

Remove head towel and use dryer to dry hair.

Comb and set hair.

Remove and clean equipment.

YOU NEED

low chair or stool

2 large pitchers of warm water (100°F)

shampoo

cotton to plug ears

pail

small plastic sheet

large rubber or plastic sheet

pillow in a plastic case

washcloth

2 bath towels

bath blanket

face towel

1 safety pin

hand hair dryer

YOU DO THIS

Check the room for drafts and warmth.

Place the chair or stool at the bedside near the head.

Cover the chair or stool seat with the small plastic sheet.

Put the pail on the covered stool.

Lower the bed to flat position.

Remove the pillow from under the patient's head.

Put on the bath blanket.

Position the patient on her back crosswise in the bed and with her head close to the edge of the bed where you stand.

Put the plastic-covered pillow under the patient's shoulders, so that the head is lower than the shoulders.

Place one bath towel around the patient's neck and pin it.

Roll three sides of the large plastic sheet to form barriers against the water.

Position the rolled plastic sheet under the patient's head so that the head is surrounded by the rolls and the ends fall over the bedside and into the pail.

Adjust the patient's head so that it hangs well within the rolled plastic sheet and slightly over the side of the bed.

Plug the patient's ears with cotton.

Give the patient the washcloth to hold over eyes.

Pour warm water over the patient's head until hair is wet. Pour gently to prevent splashing. Keep the flow away from the face.

Pour part of the shampoo onto the head, being careful not to apply any to the face.

Massage the scalp with both of your hands, using your fingertips but not your nails.

Rinse the hair well.

Apply shampoo again.

Rinse again.

Wring the patient's hair gently.

Dry the patient's forehead with the face towel and then wrap it around the patient's hair to absorb some wetness.

Lift the patient's wrapped head and remove the rolled plastic. Place it in the pail.

Pull the pillow out from under the patient's shoulders and put it under the patient's wrapped head.

Remove the face towel from the hair and replace it with a clean bath towel.

Squeeze the hair in the folds of the towel and gently rub the hair to dry.

When that towel is damp, unpin the towel from around the patient's neck, remove the damp head towel and replace it with the neck towel.

Continue rubbing and squeezing until most of the water is removed from the hair.

Use the hand dryer to finish the drying process.

Comb and set the patient's hair as desired. (*See* "Combing a Patient's Hair" in this chapter.)

Remove the plastic-covered pillow and replace with the usual pillow and case.

Report any unusual observations you made during the shampoo.

YOU NEED

a comb and brush

a towel

hair oil, a petroleum jelly such as Vaseline, or alcohol, if needed

YOU DO THIS

Spread the towel around the patient's shoulders.

Take up a few strands of hair near the scalp.

If the hair is very tangled, apply hair oil, petroleum jelly, or alcohol to these strands with gauze squares.

Wind the strands about the first finger of your left hand.

Use the comb with your right hand. Comb the ends first. Then comb further and further up the strands, letting your left finger absorb any pulls from the comb.

Repeat the procedure until all the hair is combed.

If hair is very matted, it may be necessary to cut it. Tell the charge nurse. A permission slip, signed by the patient or a member of the patient's family, may be needed before cutting.

EVENING CARE

This care should be given to all patients at night before they retire. It should be given to all bed patients in the late afternoon as well as at night.

YOU NEED

same equipment as for morning care

gown or pajamas

clean drawsheet, if bed patient

YOU DO THIS

See that the patient urinates.

See that the patient bathes his face and hands.

See that the patient has oral hygiene.

Help the patient into bed.

Wash the patient's back (if a bed patient).

Rub the patient's back with lotion.

Straighten the bed clothing. Put a clean drawsheet on the bed, if needed.

Check the unit to see that the patient's water glass and tissues are within his reach and that his bell and light switch are at his hand.

Position the bed as flat as allowed.

Remove extra pillows, if desired.

Put an extra blanket on the bed, if needed.

Raise bed side rails

Provide air and a lower room temperature.

Put the patient's used day clothing away.

Set out the patient's clothing for the next day.

Store adaptive equipment in a safe place.

14

YOUR GERIATRIC PATIENT NEEDS BOWEL AND BLADDER CONTROL

STUDY GUIDE

Tell fifteen ways in which aging can affect digestion and bowel movements.

Tell twelve ways in which aging can affect urination.

How can changes in bowel and bladder habits be noticed?

What may a patient require for help with a bowel problem?

What may a patient require for help with a urinary problem?

What do you need to offer a bedpan to a helpless patient?

Tell how to give a bedpan to a helpless patient.

Tell how to remove the bedpan.

How can you encourage a person to urinate?

What is a commode? How is it used?

What is a toilet grab bar?

Soapsuds Enema (SSE)

What is an enema?

Why is the temperature of enema water very important for a geriatric patient?

What temperature should enema water be?

What do you need in order to give an SSE?

In what position should the patient be when he is given an SSE?

How should the rectal tube be inserted into the anus?

How far should it be inserted?

If the anus is lax, how can you help prevent the enema fluid from leaking?

What should you do if a patient protests that he cannot take or hold more fluid?

What should you do when you have finished giving the enema?

What should you report for charting?

What is a Fleet enema? How is it given?

Tell how to give a rectal suppository.

Colostomy Irrigation

What is a colostomy?

What is a colostomy bag?

What do you need in order to irrigate a colostomy?

Tell how to irrigate a colostomy using a douche bag.

Tell how to irrigate a colostomy using a bulb syringe.

Removal of Feces by Digital Stimulation

What is a fecal impaction?

What happens to the patient who develops a fecal impaction?

What do you need in order to remove a fecal impaction?

In what position should the patient be for the procedure?

How do you protect the bed and genitals?

Tell how the index finger should be inserted into the anus.

Tell how to remove the impaction.

After the removal of an impaction, what do you report for charting?

Care for Incontinence

What is incontinence?

When does it occur?

How does the incontinent patient feel?

How should you treat the incontinent patient?

How can you organize care so that it is easiest for the patient and you?

Tell how to clean the incontinent bed patient.

After giving care for incontinence, what do you report for charting?

Care of Patient with Urinary Drainage

Foley Catheter Drainage

What is a Foley or indwelling catheter?

How and by whom is a Foley catheter inserted?

How is the Foley catheter attached to a drainage bag?

How long can a Foley catheter remain in a patient?

What are the dangers of Foley catheter use?

At what 3 places does infection often start when a Foley catheter is used?

Give 11 ways to help prevent urinary infection in the patient with a Foley catheter.

Condom Urinary Drainage

What is condom urinary drainage?

For whom is it ordered?

How long may a patient use the same drainage bag and rubber tubing?

How are these cared for?

How long can a patient wear the same condom?

Tell how to make a condom urinary drainage system.

Tell how to apply or change a drainage condom.

Collecting Specimens

Tell how to collect a mid-stream urine specimen.

Tell how to collect a 24-hour urine specimen.

Tell how to collect a stool specimen.

EFFECTS OF AGING

External aging is clearly visible in skin wrinkles, sagging muscles, and posture changes. Internal aging, though invisible, occurs just as surely. Age puts a constantly increasing strain on normal functioning of the internal body.

Here are some of the ways in which aging can affect normal digestion and bowel movements:

> brain damage with consequent interference with nerve impulses to the intestines
> tooth decay
> tooth abscess
> receding gums
> improperly fitted dentures
> sore tongue
> sore gums
> hernias anywhere in the system
> lowered resistance to infection anywhere in the system
> scar tissue from infections anywhere in the system
> slowdown or failure in the production of one or more enzymes or digestive juices
> cancer or other growths in the digestive system
> ulcers
> gallstones
> slowdown or failure of the bowels to move intestinal contents due to loss of muscle tone
> narrowing of a part of the intestinal tract

blockage of a part of the intestinal tract

loss of muscle tone in the anus with consequent inability to control bowel movements

varicose veins of the intestinal tract causing conditions such as hemorrhoids

Here are some of the ways in which aging can affect normal urination:

brain damage and consequent interference with the urges or abilities to drink fluids or to urinate

slowdown in the body's ability to maintain fluid balance

any body disease (even a cold) that puts a strain on the kidneys

kidney disease

kidney stones

lowered resistance to infection anywhere along the urinary system

blockage in any part of the tubes

narrowing in any part of the tubes

cancer or other growths in any part of the urinary system

pressure on the kidneys or bladder from other enlarged or misplaced abdominal organs

the effects of medication necessary for other health problems

enlargement of the prostate gland in the male

hernia in the bladder wall

loss of tone in the muscle that controls the flow of urine from the bladder

DETECTING AND HANDLING BOWEL AND BLADDER PROBLEMS

(It is very important then that all nursing personnel expect and watch for changes in the eating, drinking, urinating, and bowel moving of a geriatric patient.)

Checks of fluid and food intake at meals and times of other nourishment and daily checks of bowel movements and urinary output should be routine for all patients. Changes should be reported at once to the charge nurse, who in turn reports them to the doctor. Then the doctor orders what is necessary to correct the problem.

For bowel problems, one or more of the following may be needed:

a change in diet

medication (laxative, antacid)

a change in the patient's activity

an enema or colostomy irrigation

a suppository

removal of feces by digital stimulation

care for incontinence

For urinary problems, one or more of the following may be needed:

increased fluid intake

measured intake and output

indwelling catheter urinary drainage

condom urinary drainage

care for incontinence

GIVING A BEDPAN OR URINAL

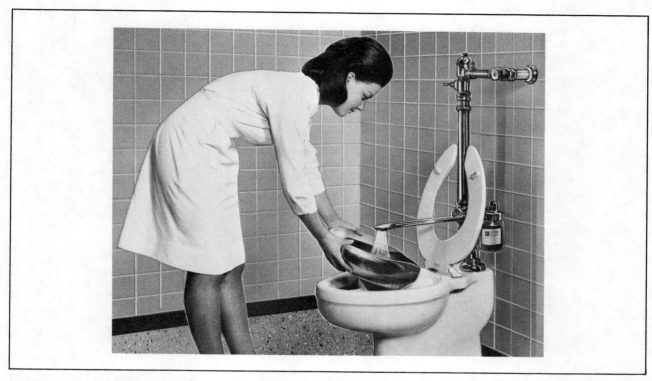

Figure 49.   A bedpan flusher on toilet. (By permission of © American Sterilizer Corp.)

Giving a Bedpan to a Helpless Patient

YOU NEED

    toilet paper

    disposable moist tissue wipers or basin of warm water and cloth

    bedpan

    bedpan cover

    5 pillows

    2 sandbags with covers

    bath blanket

    towel

YOU DO THIS

Level the mattress.

Put the bath blanket on the bed and fanfold the covers to the foot of the bed.

Go to the far side of the bed.

Raise the side rail.

Prop the pillows upright against the rail.

Return to the other side of the bed.

Move the patient close to the edge of the bed and turn him on his side toward you.

Place two of the pillows at his shoulder level. Cross the tops of these pillows so that they form an angle.

Center one pillow lengthwise beneath the crossed pillows in line with the length of the patient's spine.

Position the bedpan at the base of the lengthwise pillow so that it is aligned with the patient's buttocks.

Roll the patient back onto the pillows and bedpan.

Flex the patient's knees.

Fold the last pillow lengthwise, and slip the roll beneath the patient's knees.

Position the patient's feet together with soles flat against the mattress.

Place a sandbag on either side of the patient's feet.

To Remove the Pan

Remove the sandbags and the knee pillow.

Roll the patient toward you.

Clean the patient with toilet paper.

Wash the patient with moist tissue or warm water.

Dispose of papers into the bedpan unless fluid should be measured or a specimen obtained.

Remove the pan and place it on the bedside chair.

Remove the pillows.

Roll the patient onto his back.

Pull up the bedclothes and remove the bath blanket.

A special smaller pan can be used for patients who are difficult to handle.

Sometimes a patient has a problem starting to urinate. The urge can be stimulated by the sound of running water. Turning on a faucet or pouring water from one glass to another is usually effective. Slowly pouring lukewarm water over the genitals while the patient is on the bedpan, commode, or toilet is also effective.

THE COMMODE

A commode is an armed chair with an open seat that is higher than the one on a regular toilet (Fig. 50). A removable container attaches beneath the commode seat. It is easier for a patient to transfer to a commode than to a toilet, and the commode gives better body support. The commode can be placed beside the bed or sitting chair and the patient transferred directly onto it. After using the commode, the patient is wiped clean and returned to bed or sitting chair. The commode container is removed, emptied, and cleaned in the same way as a bedpan. Disposable containers can be used on some commodes.

TOILET GRAB BARS

Most toilets in a geriatric facility are equipped with grab bars (Fig. 51). These are waist high, strong, bent metal arms, placed one on each side of the toilet, so that the patient can support himself during the frequent insecurity of positioning himself on the toilet. Such bars make it possible for more ambulatory and wheelchair patients to use a regular toilet, although some may require your help in transferring to and from the toilet.

GIVING ENEMAS

An enema is the direction of a stream of fluid through the anus and into the rectum and large intestine. An enema is always ordered by the doctor. The kind of enema, the fluid or solution, and, sometimes, the quantity of fluid are part of the doctor's order. The doctor may order an enema for several reasons.

He may order a cleansing enema, such as SSE or Fleet, if the patient has not moved his bowels for a day or so.

He may order a tap water enema until the returns are clear to prepare a patient for x-rays of the intestines.

He may order a Fleet mineral oil enema to be retained to soften hard feces blocking the rectum.

He may order medication to be given by enema. (*See* Your Geriatric Patient Needs Medication and Inhalation Therapy.)

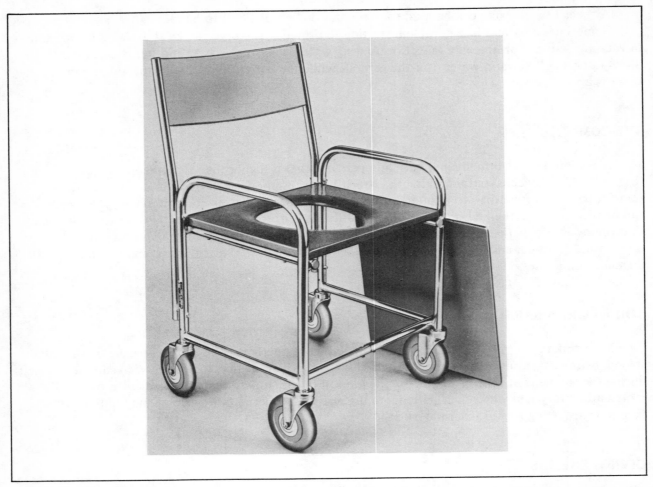

Figure 50.   A combination commode and shower chair. (Reprinted by permission of © J. A. Preston Corp., 1971.)

Soapsuds Enemas (SSE)

The temperature of the enema solution is very important. The geriatric patient cannot tolerate as much heat as the normal adult patient. If the fluid is too hot it can burn the patient. If the enema is too cold, it will not effectively stimulate bowel movement. For a geriatric patient, it should never be hotter than 105°F.

If the doctor does not specify the amount of solution, this can be determined by the condition and tolerance of the patient. A very ill patient is not given so much fluid that it causes strain or weakness. A person whose bowel is very distended with feces is unable to accept a large amount of fluid. In a geriatric patient the anus often is lax and does not retain the fluid. Gently squeezing the buttocks around the enema tube and anus may allow more inflow. As an alternative, gently pressing a sanitary napkin against the anus during the inflow can increase the amount of retained fluid.

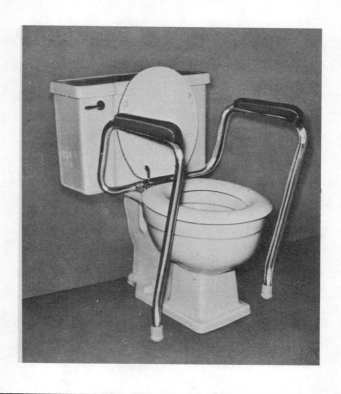

Figure 51.   Grab bars on a toilet. (Reprinted by permission of © J. A. Preston Corp., 1971.)

YOU NEED

a standard on which to hang the container of solution

1 cup to 1½ quarts of water at 105°F

liquid soap (1 ounce of soap to 1 pint of water)

enema can or bag with rubber tubing and tubing clamp

adapter to join tubes

rectal tube

lubricant, such as Vaseline

emesis basin

bedpan and toilet paper

small wash basin with warm water

washcloth and towel

disposable bed pads

YOUR GERIATRIC PATIENT NEEDS BOWEL AND BLADDER CONTROL

YOU DO THIS

Adjust the standard hook to 12 or 18 inches above the patient's hips.

Hang the can of solution.

Turn the patient onto his left side with his left arm behind his back and his right knee drawn high and relaxed on the bed. This is the Sims's position.

Protect bed with bed pads positioned under buttocks.

Fasten the rectal tube onto the container tube and adapter.

Lubricate the rectal tube.

Unclamp the tubing to expel any air in the tube. Let it drain into the emesis basin.

Reclamp the tubing and insert the rectal tube into the anus using a gentle rotating motion.

Insert for 3 or 4 inches and hold in place.

Tell the patient to relax and take deep breaths through his mouth.

Unclamp the tube and allow the solution to flow until the patient has taken all of it or until the patient protests.

If the patient protests, pinch the tube for a second or two to stop the flow and allow the patient to rest. Release the tube and lower the bag so that the fluid runs more slowly.

Watch patient for weakness or chill and end the enema if such occurs.

When finished, pinch the rectal tube near the anus and withdraw the tube slowly.

Clamp the tube and let any remaining fluid run into the emesis basin.

Disconnect the rectal tube from the adapter.

Put the rectal tube in the emesis basin.

Cover the patient and ask him to stay in Sims's position 5 or 10 minutes or as long as possible.

When the patient is ready, help him onto the bedpan.

Elevate the head of the bed if permitted and desired.

Be sure the patient has the signal bell.

Leave the patient to expel the enema.

When the enema is expelled, remove the bedpan.

If the patient wipes himself, let him wash his hands in the basin of warm water.

If you wipe the patient, have him turn on his side again and you use toilet paper and then the basin of warm water and a cloth to cleanse him.

Make the patient comfortable.

Remove the equipment from the bedside. Empty the bedpan.

Observe and chart the returns.

Clean the equipment and sterilize anything that needs such.

MEETING YOUR GERIATRIC PATIENT'S NEEDS

Oil or Retention Enema

Use a small-sized rectal tube and the amount of oil or fluid ordered. Follow the same procedure as with the SSE but attach the rectal tube to a funnel and hold the funnel 6 inches above the anus. The patient does not expel the enema but retains it. The enema is usually given at body temperature (99^6).

Clear or Tap Water Enema

Follow the same procedure as for the SSE. Repeat the procedure until the returns are clear.

Fleet Enemas

These are commercial, prepackaged, disposable enemas. There are two kinds. One is a cleansing enema and the other is an oil retention enema. The cleansing enema comes in two sizes — adult and child. These enemas are very popular because they are convenient and comfortable for both the patient and the person giving the enema. This is particularly true for the geriatric patient who cannot retain much fluid and the geriatric patient who is prone to constipation and fecal impaction. (The feces harden and pack in the rectum and lower bowel so that the patient cannot expel the mass. *See* "Fecal Impaction.")

Remove the rectal tube from the anus.

Replace the shield on the rectal tube.

Throw the squeeze bottle with the tube into the waste container.

Have the patient retain the enema as long as possible. (Since very little fluid is given in a Fleet enema, the patient may retain the enema much longer than an SSE, sometimes for several hours).

The mineral oil enema is given in the same way.

Report for charting as with an SSE.

GIVING A RECTAL SUPPOSITORY

A rectal suppository is always ordered by the doctor.

Rectal suppositories are small cones of glycerine, cocoa butter, soap, or other such easily melted substances. A cone is put through the anus and into the rectum.

Cones may be plain or medicated. Because they melt easily, they are always kept in the refrigerator.

Often one is given to stimulate bowel function or soften a hard mass of feces. Sometimes one is given to be retained and its medicine quickly absorbed into the blood stream by the many blood vessels around the anus.

YOU NEED

    the suppository

    a rubber glove or finger cot

    lubricant

YOU DO THIS

    Follow the general rules for treatments.

    Place the patient in Sims's position.

    Put on the glove.

    Lubricate the first or index finger.

    Use the finger to massage the anus and relax it.

MEETING YOUR GERIATRIC PATIENT'S NEEDS

Hold the suppository between the thumb and index finger.

Separate the buttocks with the other hand.

Insert the suppository gently into the anus.

Push it well past the anus by inserting the tip of your index finger. If the anus is lax, press a sanitary napkin against it and hold for at least ten minutes.

YOU REPORT FOR CHARTING

The time the suppository was given.

The name of the suppository.

How the patient accepted the suppository.

The results of the suppository on the patient.

COLOSTOMY

In this operation a new opening of the large intestine is surgically created on the surface of the abdomen (Fig. 52). Then the patient's bowels no longer move in the normal way but through this opening. The opening is called a stoma. The patient has no control of his bowel movements through the stoma.

Colostomy Bag

This is a small disposable plastic bag with an adhesive cuff. The bag is placed over the stoma and the cuff adheres to the skin area around the stoma. Then any fecal material is caught in the bag. The bag can be changed whenever necessary. Tincture of benzoin is sometimes put on the skin area around the stoma to toughen the skin and to help the cuff adhere well. Special odor-control tablets are available for use in the bag. A small pinprick near the top of the bag is recommended for patients who expel a great deal of gas.

Colostomy Irrigation Using a Douche Bag or Enema Can

It is necessary to irrigate a colostomy every two to three days or as the doctor orders. To irrigate means to flush or wash. Special equipment is available for this procedure and, since the treatment is repeated many times, each patient usually has his own equipment. It consists of an elastic waist belt with a hard, clear plastic bubble that fits over the stoma. The bubble has a small hole through which the irrigating catheter can be inserted into the colostomy opening. A length of disposable plastic tubing can be secured to the bottom of the bubble. The patient sits on the toilet with the tubing between his legs so that it drains into the toilet.

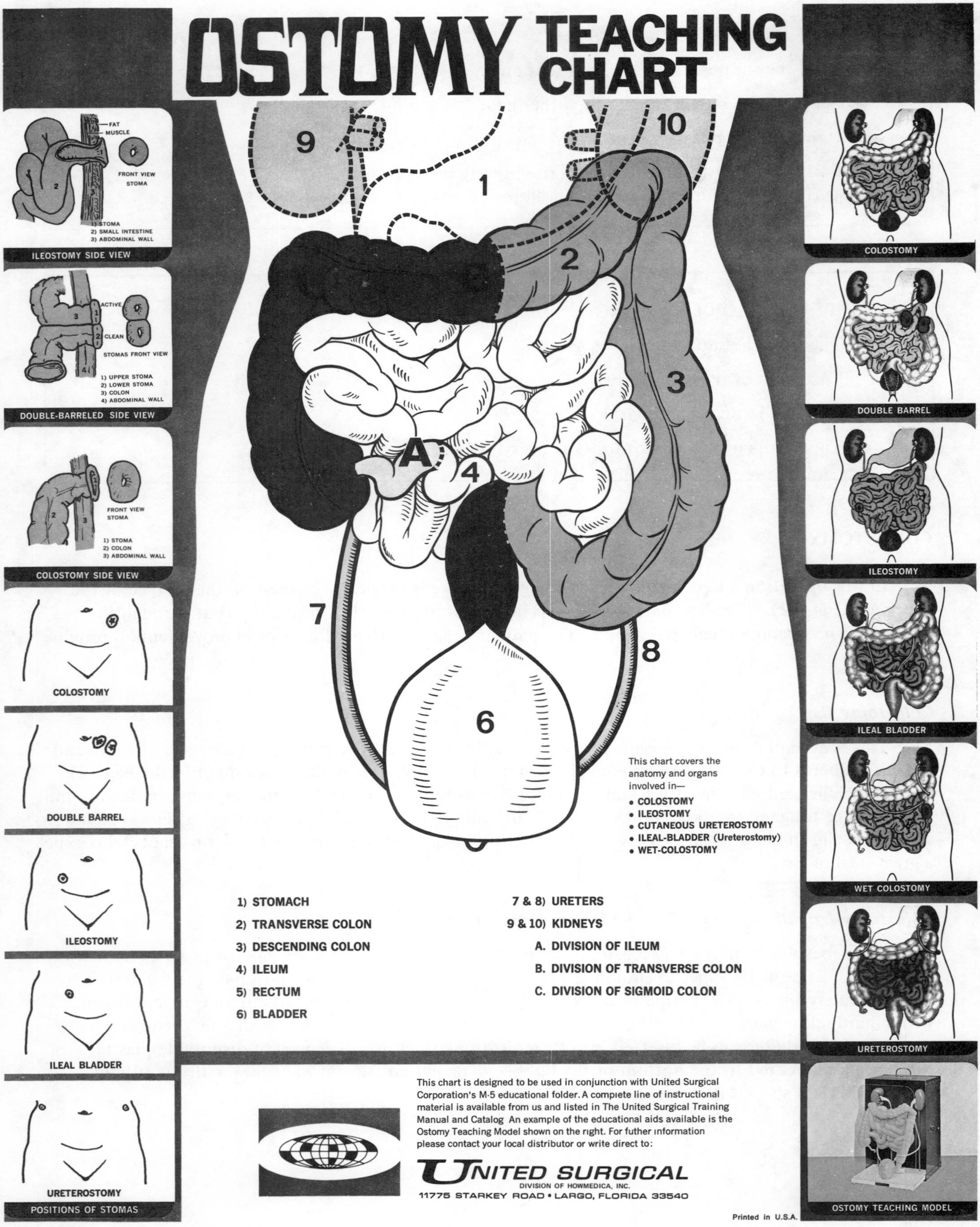
OSTOMY TEACHING CHART
FAT
MUSCLE
FRONT VIEW
STOMA
1) STOMA
2) SMALL INTESTINE
3) ABDOMINAL WALL
ILEOSTOMY SIDE VIEW
ACTIVE
CLEAN
STOMAS FRONT VIEW
1) UPPER STOMA
2) LOWER STOMA
3) COLON
4) ABDOMINAL WALL
DOUBLE-BARRELED SIDE VIEW
FRONT VIEW
STOMA
1) STOMA
2) COLON
3) ABDOMINAL WALL
COLOSTOMY SIDE VIEW
COLOSTOMY
DOUBLE BARREL
ILEOSTOMY
ILEAL BLADDER
URETEROSTOMY
POSITIONS OF STOMAS
COLOSTOMY
DOUBLE BARREL
ILEOSTOMY
ILEAL BLADDER
WET COLOSTOMY
URETEROSTOMY
OSTOMY TEACHING MODEL
This chart covers the anatomy and organs involved in—
• COLOSTOMY
• ILEOSTOMY
• CUTANEOUS URETEROSTOMY
• ILEAL-BLADDER (Ureterostomy)
• WET-COLOSTOMY
1) STOMACH
2) TRANSVERSE COLON
3) DESCENDING COLON
4) ILEUM
5) RECTUM
6) BLADDER
7 & 8) URETERS
9 & 10) KIDNEYS
A. DIVISION OF ILEUM
B. DIVISION OF TRANSVERSE COLON
C. DIVISION OF SIGMOID COLON
This chart is designed to be used in conjunction with United Surgical Corporation's M-5 educational folder. A complete line of instructional material is available from us and listed in The United Surgical Training Manual and Catalog An example of the educational aids available is the Ostomy Teaching Model shown on the right. For futher information please contact your local distributor or write direct to:
UNITED SURGICAL
DIVISION OF HOWMEDICA, INC.
11775 STARKEY ROAD • LARGO, FLORIDA 33540
Printed in U.S.A.

Figure 52. Types of "ostomies." (By permission of © United Surgical Co.)

YOU NEED

colostomy irrigation set of belt, bubble, and sheath (disposable irrigating tubing)

douche bag or can

1—2 quarts of warm water

lubricant

adapter

small-sized catheter

clean colostomy bag

tincture of benzoin

cotton-tipped applicator

YOU DO THIS

Sit patient on toilet.

Apply colostomy bubble, belt, and sheath.

Use the adapter to attach the catheter to the douche bag tubing.

Hold the douche bag or can 12 to 18 inches above the stoma.

Clear the air from the tubing by letting some water run through it.

Pinch the catheter near the end.

Lubricate the catheter tip.

Insert the catheter through the bubble opening and then into the stoma 6 to 8 inches. Use care.

Allow the water to run in. The water runs out almost at once and drains through the disposable tubing into the toilet. The water loosens and carries the feces with it.

After the water has run in, remove the catheter.

Allow the patient to remain on the toilet for 15 to 20 minutes.

Remove and dispose of the plastic tubing.

Remove the belt and bubble.

Clean the stoma and the skin area around it. Dry the skin area.

Apply tincture of benzoin to the skin area.

Use scissors to shape the opening of the colostomy bag to the size of the stoma.

Apply the colostomy bag around the stoma to skin area.

Help the patient off the toilet and make him comfortable.

Clean the irrigation set and ready it for the next irrigation.

Observe and chart the results of the treatment.

If the patient is not allowed bathroom privileges, the irrigation may be done at his bed. The patient may either sit on the side of the bed or lie in a comfortable position. The belt is put on and the bubble placed over the stoma. One end of the disposable tubing is secured to the bubble and the other end placed in a bedpan at the bedside. Remember to follow the general rules for all treatments.

Since privacy is normal and helpful during bowel movements, the patient is usually taught to irrigate his colostomy, to change colostomy bags, and to care for the stoma. But when he is weak, confused, or otherwise unable, you must do it.

Report for charting as with an SSE.

Colostomy Irrigation Using a Bulb Syringe

Instead of a bag and catheter, a bulb syringe tipped with a piece of flexible rubber tubing or plastic tubing is used.

YOU NEED

    colostomy belt, bubble, and sheath

    bulb syringe with rubber or plastic tubing tip

    disposable plastic tubing

    pitcher with 24 oz. of water at 105°F.

    lubricant

YOU DO THIS

    Apply the colostomy bubble, belt, and sheath.

    Squeeze the bulb syringe to remove air before inserting the tip in water.

    Draw water into the syringe.

    Hold the tip of the syringe upward and press the bulb to remove remaining air.

    Draw more water into the syringe.

    Lubricate the tip and insert into the stoma for 3 to 5 inches.

    Hold with the bulb up. Use both your thumbs to compress it, so that water flows in a steady stream.

Refill the bulb as necessary.

Avoid putting air into the stoma.

Have the patient take long, deep breaths during the irrigation.

Have the patient massage the area around the stoma during the irrigation.

Allow patient to remain on toilet for 15 or 20 minutes after irrigation.

After removing the sheath, clean the stoma and attach a clean colostomy bag.

When discharge ceases, remove the bag, clean the stoma, and cover it with a gauze dressing spread with lubricant. This can be held in place by an elastic girdle, shorts, or a clean colostomy bag. This dressing is used when stoma or skin is irritated.

Report for charting as with an SSE.

FECAL IMPACTION

Feces that are allowed to remain in the lower bowel and rectum become hard and packed, and the patient finds it impossible to expel the stool.

When this occurs, the patient becomes ill. He may lose his appetite, experience nausea, vomit, have a fever, have chills, sweat, experience stomach cramps and other discomforts. His abdomen may swell and become hard. Sometimes he appears to have diarrhea, but it is only liquid seeping through the hard mass of impacted stool. There is only one thing to be done for this patient. The impacted feces must be removed by stimulation of the bowel with the index or first finger.

Some geriatric patients are susceptible to fecal impaction. If a patient's bowels do not respond well to the usual means of regulation ordered by the doctor (that is: diet, sufficient fluids, medications, enemas, suppositories), then the doctor may order removal of stools by digital stimulation. He usually orders a mineral oil enema or suppository to precede the digital stimulation by 15 or 20 minutes.

Digital (Finger) Stimulation to Remove Rectal Feces

YOU NEED

bedpan and cover

toilet tissue

disposable bed pads

sanitary napkins

2 or more pairs of disposable gloves

lubricating jelly

basin of warm water and soap

towel

disposable washcloth

plastic disposable bag

YOU DO THIS

Position the patient on his left side with his right knee drawn up (Sims's position).

Place the disposable bed pads well under the patient's buttocks.

Cover the genitals with a sanitary napkin.

Place the bedpan on the bed near the disposable pads.

Put on disposable gloves and apply lubricating jelly to your index or forefinger.

Massage the anus with that finger. Put more jelly on the finger and insert it gently into the rectum, directing it slowly upward and toward the patient's spine. Work the finger around the packed feces, loosening the mass gently and pulling it toward the anus.

Put the bedpan in position to catch the fecal mass as it is removed.

Change gloves when needed, discarding them into the plastic bag.

Apply lubricant as often as needed.

Remove as much feces as possible, being careful to prevent injury or bleeding. (When the rectal part of the impaction is removed, the rest often is naturally expelled).

When finished, clean the bed and clean and wash the patient.

Position him comfortably.

Put a disposable bed pad under his buttocks.

Straighten the bedclothes.

Remove, clean, and put away equipment.

REPORT FOR CHARTING

The time of the removal.

How it was accepted by the patient.

The color, consistency, odor, and amount of feces removed, and the presence of mucus, blood, or other material.

The effect of the removal on the patient.

Example: A large, hard mass of feces about the size of an orange was broken up and removed by digital stimulation. The feces were very dark greenish brown, and there were several streaks of thick white mucus. The patient was cooperative and felt weak but relieved after the removal.

THE INCONTINENT PATIENT

Common reactions of patients to incontinence are nervousness, disgust, anger, and depression. The patient may cry, moan, insist that he wants to die, scream, use abusive language, refuse to eat, demand constant attention, and refuse to cooperate or to take part in any activities.

Sometimes this kind of behavior seems willful and is exasperating to busy nursing personnel, and they may be tempted to ignore the patient, to avoid him as much as possible, to hurry through any necessary care, and to separate him from other patients who might be annoyed by him.

Nothing could be worse for the incontinent patient. Even if he is given the best of physical care, such neglect and isolation are so psychologically harmful that they can destroy the patient's will to live.

Instead, this patient needs more attention. He needs understanding, respect, and affection. He needs to be reassured that:

    he is liked and accepted by others.
    incontinence is not shameful.
    incontinence can happen to anyone.
    incontinence can be managed with a minimum of discomfort, embarrassment and time.
    an incontinent patient can lead a good, happy life.

In a nursing facility, discussion of the patient during staff meetings and evaluations of patients allow the staff to develop a plan of nursing care that meets both the physical and the psychological needs of this patient. Such a plan might include the following:

    visiting with the patient at times when he doesn't need changing or other nursing care.
    including the patient in as many group activities as possible.
    encouraging the patient to talk about his incontinence and how he can help with managing it.
    instituting a toilet retraining program.
    finding out the patient's interests and discussing them during changing times.
    organizing the changing process so that it is a quick, simple procedure.
    giving special attention such as an extra dessert or a flower by the bedside. Such attention
        however, should be given freely and never as a reward for bowel and bladder control
        or his cooperation.

⟨ *Retraining the Incontinent Patient* ⟩

Retraining a patient to control bowel and bladder function is desirable because it allows the patient to lead a more normal life. Retraining is not always possible, however, and when possible it is often a long, difficult, and discouraging process that cannot be successful without the enthusiastic cooperation of patient and all shifts of nursing personnel.

A retraining program should be the outgrowth of an evaluation of the patient that includes an understanding of his specific physical, psychological, and social needs and capabilities. This knowledge should also determine the right moment for starting the program.

The program and procedure must be explained fully to the patient and to all shifts of nursing personnel.

Regular progress reports and suggestions by the patient and nursing personnel are needed to sustain interest in the program.

Any program should include the following:

adequate diet.

frequent offerings of drinking water and other fluids.

use of a sitting position regardless of whether the retraining is with a toilet, commode, or bedpan. (Bowel and bladder cannot empty completely when a person is lying down, as shown in Fig. 53.)

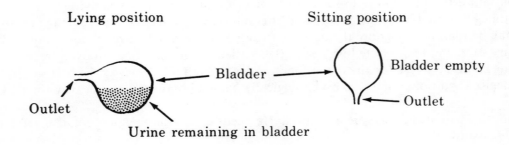

Figure 53. Relation of bladder emptying to patient's position. (From Elementary Rehabilitation Nursing Care, U.S. Public Health Service, Division of Nursing.)

discussion with the patient about his normal bowel and bladder habits and observation of his pattern of incontinence.

based on his habits and pattern, a daily 24-hour schedule and record sheet that specifies the times for 20 minutes of toileting at every two-hour interval. (Once control is established, the schedule can be changed to every three or four hours.)

the faithful carrying out of the schedule with no exceptions allowed.

the help and encouragement of nursing personnel during positioning and toileting.

a plan of physical exercise to stimulate and regulate bowel and bladder functions.

a plan of mental activity to distract the patient from thinking about himself.

use of items between toileting that prevent bed soiling, such as adult diapers, sanitary napkins, and shower caps filled with disposable tissues or gauze.

setting an alarm clock for the night schedule.

dressing the patient in street clothes during the day.

selecting street clothing that allows easy toileting.

YOU NEED

basin of warm water

soap

disposable washcloths

disposable gloves

bath towels

newspaper or large piece of disposable plastic

disposable bag

toilet tissue

clean bed sheets (as needed)

disposable bed pads

clean gown

air deodorizer

YOU DO THIS

See that the room is warm and free of drafts.

Collect everything needed on the bedside table.

Draw the curtain around the patient's bed.

Level the mattress.

Tell the patient what you are going to do.

Remove the spread and blanket from the bed.

(*See* Making an Occupied Bed.)

Spread the newspaper on the floor.

Loosen the top sheet.

Remove the patient's gown and put it on the newspaper.

Go to the far side of the bed.

Move the patient to the side of the bed that you are facing.

(*See* Your Patient Needs Sleep, Rest, Positioning, and Transferring.)

Turn the patient so that he faces you.

Raise the side rail on the bed.

Return to the other side of the bed.

Spread open the disposable bag. (The bag can be placed into the patient's wastepaper container and the bag top cuffed over the top of the container.)

Put on disposable gloves.

Turn back the top sheet to expose the patient's back, buttocks, and thighs.

Use toilet tissue to remove as much of the feces as possible from the patient's body and the bed sheets. Discard into the disposable bag.

Loosen the drawsheet and fold it so that a clean part is under the patient. Then roll the sheet against the patient's back.

Wet a disposable washcloth and remove the feces from the patient's body. Discard that cloth.

Use another washcloth to clean the patient thoroughly with soap and water. Rinse off all soap. Dry the patient.

Use the same washcloth and soap and water to clean the plastic drawsheet. Dry the sheet thoroughly.

Cover the roll of soiled drawsheet with a disposable bed pad.

Put a clean drawsheet (and bottom sheet, if needed) on that side of the bed.

Roll the patient to the clean side of the bed.

Raise the bed rail.

Go to the other side of the bed.

Lower the side rail.

Remove the soiled sheets from that side of the bed. Put them on the newspapers.

Wash and dry any part of the patient that is soiled.

Wash and dry any soiled part of the plastic sheet.

Make the bottom sheets on that side of the bed.

Rub the patient's back, buttocks, and thighs with skin lotion.

Notice any redness or rash.

Position the patient on his back.

Check the genitals to see that all areas are clean.

Return to the other side of the bed.

Lower the bed rail.

Change the disposable bed pad.

Put a clean gown on the patient.

Make the top of the bed.

Position the patient comfortably.

Use air deodorizer.

Remove the soiled laundry in the newspaper.

Remove all equipment. Clean, sanitize, and put away the patient's basin.

Follow the procedure for soiled linen. (Some nursing facilities soak soiled linen before sending it to the laundry.)

Report to the charge nurse the amount, color, and consistency of the bowel movement and any change in the patient's skin.

CARE OF PATIENTS WITH URINARY DRAINAGE

A doctor may order urinary drainage for a patient who is unable to control urinary flow. For female patients, and sometimes for males, the doctor orders indwelling catheter urinary drainage. For other males, the doctor orders condom urinary drainage.

Foley or Indwelling Catheter Drainage

The Foley catheter is a soft rubber catheter with a small, inflatable balloon on the insertion tip. The catheter is inserted into the bladder under sterile conditions by a doctor or professional nurse. The balloon is then inflated. This prevents the catheter from slipping out of the bladder.

The catheter is attached to sterile, disposable, plastic tubing (Fig. 54), and the end of the tubing is inserted into a sterile drainage bag. Several types of drainage bags are used. One type is attached to the side of the bed. Another type is fastened onto the patient's leg.

A Foley catheter can remain in a patient for several days.

Urinary Infection

Because an indwelling catheter irritates the membranes of the urethra and bladder, the patient is subject to urinary infection. Every effort to prevent such infection must be made through the careful attention of all nursing personnel. Your specific responsibilities as an aide, in the care of patients with indwelling catheters, may differ from one nursing facility to another. Every nursing care plan, however, includes most of the precautions to be discussed here. Do not touch any part of an indwelling catheter drainage system unless you have been instructed in your specific duties as an aide. If any part of a drainage system does not appear to be in correct position or working well, report to the charge nurse at once.

Where Infections Often Start

around the catheter where it enters the body.
on the end of the drainage tube that is inserted into the drainage bag.
at the point where the catheter and drainage tube join.

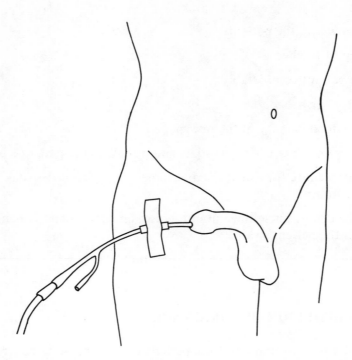

Figure 54. Positioning and taping of penis with indwelling catheter. (By permission of New York University Medical Center, Department of Rehabilitative Medicine.)

General Rules for Preventing Urinary Infection

Encourage the patient to drink plenty of fluids. Most patients with indwelling catheters are on measured intake and output and are expected to drink at least 3000 cc. of fluid daily. (*See* Your Geriatric Patient Needs Food and Fluid Balance.)

Prevent pull on the catheter by looping the drainage tube. Secure the loop to the bed by passing an elastic band around the tube and pinning the elastic to the drawsheet.

Watch the drainage tube and drainage bag to see that urine is flowing freely. Take special notice:
> when turning, dressing, or positioning a patient.
> just after the catheter is attached to the drainage tube.
> just after the catheter is inserted in the drainage tube.

Irrigate the bladder regularly with sterile solution. (This should always be done by a professional nurse.) After bladder irrigation, flush the drainage tube with the irrigating solution. If the tube is not clean after flushing, discard it and connect a new sterile tube.

If the catheter and tubing are detached, as for irrigation, put a sterile cap over the tube end. To reattach the catheter, remove the cap from the tube and wipe the tube tip with an anteseptic swab.

Empty any drainage bag before it is three-fourths full. An overly full bag can cause urine to back up in the drainage tube.

Do not allow the tube end that enters the drainage bag to come in contact with anything other than the sterile inside of the drainage bag.

On a male patient, tape the catheter to the upper thigh so that the penis lies horizontal across the thigh. Alternate the catheter taping daily between one thigh and the other. Prevent a kink in the catheter by putting a piece of plastic tubing over the catheter at the site of taping.

Clean the patient's genitals with soap and water daily and more often if needed. Since matter tends to collect under the foreskin of an uncircumcized male, gently draw back the foreskin to clean that area.

Clear away any secretion around the point at which the catheter enters the body. Report crusts or irritations to the charge nurse at once.

Wrap a gauze square dipped in Zephiran or another antiseptic solution around the tip of the penis and the catheter.

Condom Urinary Drainage

A condom is a thin rubber sheath that fits snugly over the penis, the male sex organ. The sheath is perforated at the tip which is attached to one end of a length of rubber tubing. The other end of the tube is inserted into a drainage bag.

Whenever possible, doctors order condom drainage for male patients because the dangers of urinary infection are less than when indwelling catheters are used.

Applying a condom drainage system is not a sterile procedure, but cleanliness of equipment and method is essential. A patient may use the same rubber tubing and drainage bag over a period of several months. A regular routine for cleaning and sanitizing this equipment must be followed. The patient has two sets of equipment, which are alternated. When one set is in use, the other is cleaned and sanitized

A patient may wear one condom throughout a 48-hour period. He should be checked often during every night and day, however, to see that the condom has not become twisted and that urine is draining. He should also be checked daily for signs of skin irritation or indications that the condom is no longer properly applied.

Making a Condom Urinary Drainage System (Fig. 55)

YOU NEED

    a new condom

    a piece of rubber drainage tubing.

    2 thin rubber rings made by cutting the end of a rubber tube

    straight pin

YOU DO THIS

    Slide one rubber ring over the end of the drainage tubing until it is about 1½ inches from the end.

    Hold the rolled condom so that the rolled edge is down.

    Place the condom on top of the ringed end of the drainage tube.

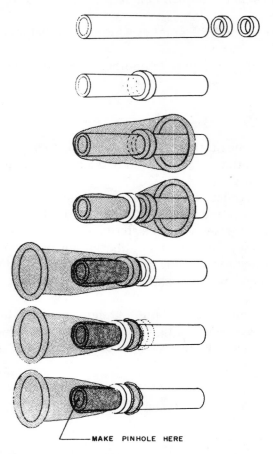

MAKE PINHOLE HERE

Figure 55. A condom urinary drainage system. (By permission of New York University Medical Center.) Basic Nursing Ward Procedure Manual: Rehabilitation Monograph.

Unroll the condom from the inside until it covers the tube and the ring. Hold it in place.

Slide the second ring over the condom-covered tube end to a distance of about 1 inch from the end.

Pull the rolled edge of the condom back over itself and the second ring.

Slide the first ring over the second ring to lock the condom in place over the tube.

Push the rolled edge of the condom below the rings to expose the condom-covered tip of the tube.

Use the straight pin to puncture a hole in the center of the condom where it covers the tip of the drainage tube.

Pull the condom back over the tip of the drainage tube so that the rolled edge is about 2 inches free from the tip of the tube.

YOU NEED

a basin of warm water

soap

a towel and washcloth

a razor

a paper towel

tincture of benzoin

cotton-tipped applicators

surgical cement

a drainage condom connected to the patient's drainage tube

a patient's urinary drainage bag

tube connectors

small gauze pads

YOU DO THIS

Wash the genital area with soap and water. Draw back the foreskin and clean beneath it.

Use the razor to remove excess pubic hair that could be caught when surgical cement is applied to the penis.

Check the skin of the penis for redness or irritation.

Report any such signs to the charge nurse before continuing.

Paint the skin of the penis with tincture of benzoin. Allow it to dry.

Make a hole in the center of the paper towel and slide it onto the penis so that the towel protects the patient's pubic hair.

Before cementing the condom in place, be sure there is about a 2-inch distance between the tip of the penis and the tip of the rubber tubing.

Starting behind the foreskin, use an applicator to encircle the skin of the penis with a succession of thin layers of surgical cement; unroll the condom after each application to cover the cemented part. Never put cement on the tip of the penis.

After the condom is cemented in place, attach the free end of the tube to an adaptor.

Screw the adaptor to the inlet of the patient's drainage bag.

If a leg drainage bag is used, fasten the leg straps either above or below the knee, whichever is most suited to the patient's needs.

Put a gauze pad between the patient's skin and any pressure point created by the bag fastenings.

COLLECTING SPECIMENS

Specimens are samples of body material or wastes that are sent to a laboratory for tests and examinations to find out whether the material is abnormal in certain respects.

Before Collecting Any Specimen

Be sure you understand how to collect the specimen. If in doubt, ask the charge nurse.
Select the right container for the specimen.
Be sure the container has a tight-fitting cover.
Make out the right laboratory report specimen sheet, or slip, and the label for the specimen.
Be sure the patient's name, room number, date, and type of specimen are on the label and the specimen sheet.

After Collecting Any Specimen

Attach the laboratory report specimen sheet to the specimen with a rubber band or clip.
Chart the kind of specimen and the time of collection.
Put the collection container in the right place for laboratory pick-up.

URINE SPECIMENS

When collecting all urine specimens, note on the label and also on the laboratory report specimen sheet if the patient has known rectal or other type of bleeding to account for blood or blood cells in urine.

Routine

Have the patient void into a bedpan or directly into an unsterile but clean urine specimen bottle.

Mid-Stream Urine

Have the patient start to void; then hold the specimen bottle to catch running urine.

Clean-Voided Urine

Clean the patient's genitals with sterile cotton balls and antiseptic solution. Then have the patient void into a sterile bedpan and transfer the urine to a sterile specimen bottle, or, after cleaning the genitals, catch a mid-stream sample in a sterile specimen bottle.

Twenty-Four-Hour Urine

Use a 1-gallon bottle.

Label the bottle with the patient's name, room number, and the hours of the collection. This bottle is usually kept in a refrigerator during the collection.

Example: Tom Jones Rm 314 9/3/69
       6:50 A.M. to 6:50 A.M. 24-hr. collection urine
      (The date marked is the one for the starting hour.)

Label the patient's bedpan in the same way.

Put the patient's name and the hours of the specimen on any collection lists in the utility or hopper room, or post a sign in his bathroom.

See that the chart is marked with the time the specimen is begun.

See that all aides and nurses are advised that the specimen is to begin.

Have the patient void just before the start of the collection period and discard that voiding. Start the collection with the next voiding. Put the exact time of the discarded voiding on the collection label. (*Example:* 6:50 A.M.)

Tell the patient that he is on a 24-hour urine collection and that he must use his bedpan or urinal whenever he needs to void.

When he wants to have a bowel movement, he must void first or afterward into his specimen pan, but he should not void during the bowel movement; otherwise he will spoil the urine collection. He should have a separate pan for bowel movements. That pan should be marked BM for bowel movement.

Add the urine from each voiding to the gallon collection bottle.

At the end of the collection time, mix the urine in the bottle and measure the full amount.

If the total amount is required in the laboratory, put the urine back in the bottle and send it to the laboratory with the right laboratory report specimen sheet.

If portions, or aliquots, of the urine are required, measure out the amounts ordered into the right bottles and send them with the right laboratory report specimen sheets to the laboratory. Then discard the remaining urine.

Be sure the laboratory report and the chart are marked with the following:

    all the information on the collection bottle label.

    the time of the last voiding that ended the specimen.

    the total amount in cc.

    what amounts were sent to the laboratory.

    what tests were to be done with each of these amounts.

STOOL SPECIMEN

Do not let the patient void into the bedpan being used to collect a stool specimen. (Use the same technique as with a 24-hour urine collection.)

Use a disposable wooden blade to transfer feces from the bedpan to the specimen container.

Do not refrigerate the specimen unless a nurse tells you to do so. Most stool specimens should not be refrigerated.

15

YOUR GERIATRIC PATIENT NEEDS MEDICATION AND INHALATION THERAPY

STUDY GUIDE

What must a pharmacist put on any prescription?

What seven important facts are included on a prescription label?

If you had to give medicine, what type of sheet would help you check all the seven important facts that appear on a label?

Tell how you would check and double-check before giving any medication.

Where should a patient's medicine be kept?

What are the usual ways of giving medications at home?

What do you need to give oral or PO medicines?

What do you need to give rectal medicines?

What do you need to give medicines to the skin?

What do you need to give medicines by injection?

How can you check medicine-taking by a geriatric patient?

Who is allowed to be in charge of his own medication?

What is inhalation therapy?

Why is tanked oxygen contained in heavy steel?

How are oxygen flow and speed of flow regulated on an oxygen tank?

Who orders oxygen?

What is included in an order for oxygen?

What is the abbreviation for oxygen?

What is an O_2 tent?

How is it used?

What is the usual rate of flow for oxygen tent use?

Why should a patient's head and shoulders be covered inside an oxygen tent?

How is a nasal catheter used to give oxygen?

Who should insert a nasal catheter?

What is the usual rate of flow used for a nasal catheter?

What is a disposable nasal cannula?

How does the nasal cannula work?

How is oxygen given by mask?

What are the safety rules for using oxygen?

Tell how to watch an oxygen tank.

Tell how to crack an oxygen tank.

Tell how to shut off an oxygen tank.

What is a Bird or a Bennet?

How does a respirator work?

When is a respirator used?

How can a respirator be used?

Name two ways by which respirator air can be delivered to a patient.

Tell how to give a steam inhalation.

Tell how to give mouth to mouth resuscitation.

ABOUT PRESCRIPTIONS

A pharmacist, or person licensed by state law to prepare and dispense medicines, fills a doctor's prescription.

Any prescription is always labeled. The label tells the following very important facts.
Patient's name
Prescription order number
Doctor's name
How the medicine is to be given (*example:* by mouth)
When the medicine is to be given (*example:* every four hours except when sleeping)
How much of the medicine is to be given at any one time (*example:* two tablets for first does, one tablet thereafter).
Whether the medicine needs special care (*example:* refrigerate).

GENERAL RULES FOR GIVING MEDICINES

Before giving a medicine check to see that you know:
The correct medicine
The correct amount
The correct time

MEETING YOUR GERIATRIC PATIENT'S NEEDS

The correct person

The correct way to give it

Make out a 24-hour medicine time sheet that lists all the patient's medicines next to the times they are to be given. Next to each, write the amount and how the medicine is to be given. Then you need only look at the sheet to know which amount of what medication your patient should take at what hour.

Example: The patient has five different medicines.

Time	Prescription Number	Amount	Directions
6:00 A.M.	#18932	1 cap.	one capsule by mouth every four hours night and day
7:30 A.M.	#26705	2 tab.	two tablets by mouth before meals three times a day
10:00 A.M.	#18932	1 cap.	as at 6:00 A.M.
10:00 A.M.	#37602	1 tab.	1 tablet by mouth every day
10:00 A.M.	#43102	1 t.	one teaspoon by mouth every morning
11:30 A.M.	#26705	2 tab.	as at 7:30 A.M.
2:00 P.M.	#18932	1 cap.	as at 6:00 A.M.
5:30 P.M.	#26705	2 tab.	as at 7:30 A.M.
6:00 P.M.	#18932	1 cap.	as at 6:00 A.M.
10:00 P.M.	#18932	1 cap.	as at 6:00 A.M.
10:00 P.M.	#23401	1 suppository	(rectal) at bedtime (refrigerate)
2:00 A.M.	#18932	1 cap.	as at 6:00 A.M.

YOU DO THIS

Check your watch with the medicine time sheet. Check the prescription number, the amount, and directions on the time sheet.

Read the complete label before opening any medicine bottle. Check the label against the time sheet information.

Pour the medicine. If it is in tablet or capsule form, shake the correct number to be given into the cap of the bottle and then use the cap to pour that number into a small, dry glass.

Read the label again before you close the medicine bottle.

Check all the information about the poured medicine again.

Close the bottle and return it to safe storage.

Take to the bedside whatever you need to give the medicine.

Check the name of the patient with the name on the medicine time sheet.

Then, give the medicine to the patient.

YOUR GERIATRIC PATIENT NEEDS MEDICATION AND INHALATION THERAPY

After giving a medicine, stay with the patient until the medicine is swallowed or otherwise taken.

Watch for and report any unusual symptom that might be a reaction to the medicine.

Report for charting or otherwise write down when the medicine was given and how the patient accepted it. Do this at once, so that there is no possibility of an extra dose being given.

TO GIVE MEDICINES AT HOME

Unless a medicine needs special care, all of the patient's medicine bottles should be kept together and apart from medicines belonging to other family members. All medicines should be out of the reach of children or animals.

Usual Ways of Giving Medicines at Home

Orally

YOU NEED

    glass of fresh water

    small glass or paper cup for the medicine

    a measure if needed

    a slice of fruit or cracker (if the medicine tastes bad)

Some medicines must be given with food. This is indicated on the label. If taken at a time other than mealtime, a glass of milk is usually given.

By Rectum

YOU NEED

    a retention enema set-up or finger cot with lubricant

To the Skin

> **YOU NEED**
>
> a set-up for whatever the treatment ordered: soaks, compresses, and so forth

By Injection

An aide must never give an injection except in unusual circumstances and under the instruction and supervision of a doctor and professional nurse.

> **YOU NEED**
>
> sterile syringes and needles of the right size (usually disposable)
>
> sterile alcohol wiper for preparing the skin

Through Inhalation

> **YOU NEED**
>
> a steam inhalator

MEDICINE-TAKING BY GERIATRIC PATIENTS

Most geriatric patients take several kinds of medicine each day. Whenever possible, doctors prefer patients to be in charge of taking their own medications. Self-medication is therefore allowed in many home care, day care and minimal care nursing home services. The following methods are useful in reminding the patient to take his medicine and in checking on whether he has done so.

Have separate containers for each kind of medicine but give the patient the amounts he will use on a daily basis. (*Example:* If his prescription instructions are for one capsule three times a day, each morning give him a container with three capsules.)

See that each container is correctly marked with prescription information.

Make out a daily 24-hour medicine time sheet for the patient to keep and to refer to. Go over the sheet with him to be sure that he understands it. Each time he takes a medicine, he can cross it off the list.

If he must take medicine at a set hour, give him an alarm clock with the alarm set for the correct time.

See that he has access to whatever he may need to take with the medicine. (*Example:* water, milk, and so forth.)

INHALATION THERAPY

Some conditions, such as heart diseases and emphysema, are treated with inhalation therapy on a doctor's orders.

Inhalation means the process of drawing air or gas into the lungs.

Tanked gases, such as oxygen and carbon dioxide, are used in inhalation therapy.

No one should give, regulate, or shut off inhalation equipment unless he is familiar with the specific order for the patient and familiar with the administration of the specific gas ordered. Many nursing homes and hospitals have inhalation departments. Workers in these departments are specially trained to administer therapeutic gases.

Of all the gases, the most commonly used is oxygen.

EQUIPMENT USED IN GIVING OXYGEN (O_2)

The O_2 Tank

Tanked oxygen is tightly contained in heavy steel that prevents the gas from escaping. A special head with two valve controls regulates the flow of oxygen and the speed of the flow. When a doctor orders oxygen, he also orders the speed at which the oxygen is to be given. His order might read: O_2 at 6 liters. (O_2 stands for oxygen.) A liter is the measuring unit of the O_2 flow.

Tanked O_2 can be given in the following ways:

> by oxygen tent
> by nasal catheter
> by nasal cannula
> by nose and mouth mask

The O_2 Tent

This is a light, movable tent made of clear plastic and attached to a special sparkproof motor-driven unit. The motor circulates and cools the air inside the tent. The usual rate of O_2 flow in a tent is 10–12 liters. A thermostat keeps the temperature within the tent at about 70°F. It is quite drafty inside the tent and the patient's head and shoulders should be protected by towels. The tent fits over the head of the bed so that the patient's head and chest are inside. The back and sides of the tent are tucked as far under the mattress as they will go.

The tent front is folded within a folded drawsheet and that sheet tucked in on either side of the bed so that no oxygen leaks out.

There are zippered openings on both sides of the tent through which patient care is given. These openings should be closed except when care is in progress.

When the bed is made, the tent is moved from one side of the bed to the other with the patient.

254

Nasal Catheter or Tube

A small catheter is inserted into the nose, by either a doctor or a nurse, and strapped with adhesive to the forehead. The catheter connects to larger tubing which connects to either a wall O_2 supply or to a tank. The flow of O_2 is usually 4–6 liters. Tubing should be pinned to the sheet near the head of the bed to prevent pull on the catheter. Secure a loop of tubing by passing an elastic band around the tube and pinning the elastic to the sheet.

Nasal Cannula

A nasal cannula for oxygen is made of plastic and is disposable. Two short tubes enter the patient's nostrils and are held in place by an adjustable strap that fits over the ears and under the chin. This is a very convenient method of administering O_2 and the patient is often able to use it himself without aid. The flow is usually 4–6 liter.

Mask

A mask fits tightly over the nose and mouth and is attached to the O_2 supply by tubing. The flow of O_2 is usually 8 liters.

SAFETY RULES FOR O_2

Danger: When pure O_2 is given, chances of fire or explosion are great. Steps must be taken to avoid disaster. Safety rules must be followed.

Post *No Smoking* signs in any room or unit where O_2 is used.

One sign is usually posted at the door or entrance and another sign is posted on the O_2 tank.

See that the patient and his visitors are warned of danger and cautioned against lighting matches.

Do not use ordinary electrical things in the area. These would include heating pads, stoves, razors, machines, and radios. Special sparkproofed equipment, such as the motor for an O_2 tent, is used when necessary.

Have the patient use a hand-rung dinner bell instead of the electric call bell.

Do not wear fabrics that cause sparks and do not allow the patient to wear them. These fabrics include wool, silk, rayon, nylon, and other synthetics.

Put cotton blankets on the bed.

WATCHING AN O_2 TANK

Before starting a new tank, check the label on the tank to be sure it is O_2 and not another gas.

Temperature changes expand and contract oxygen. To allow for such changes the meter of a tank reads to 3000, but the tank is considered full if it registers 2000. At home, a new tank should be ordered when the meter on the one in use reads 1000 or one-half full. This is because a delivery may take several days.

In a nursing facility that has an oxygen supply room a new tank should be ordered when the gauge reads 500–1000. Many institutions keep two tanks at the bedside, one in use and one filled and awaiting use. When the tank in use runs out, the spare is attached at once and a new tank is then ordered to replace the spare.

Oxygen tanks are very heavy and because of this they are delivered strapped to special carriers. While in use, a tank should remain strapped on the carrier and care should be taken to prevent dropping the tank.

The glass jar or humidifier must be kept filled with water to the measure marked on the glass. When O_2 is flowing, the water bubbles. Oxygen is very drying; bubbling it through water moistens it.

STARTING, OR CRACKING, AN O_2 TANK

A new tank must be "cracked" or opened and the "head" or part that consists of the meters, valves, and humidifier, fitted to it. This is done by trained personnel. First open the valve of the tank until the capacity amount registers on the gauge meter. Then open the liter regulator and set it at the desired reading. Both of these are right turns.

SHUTTING OFF AN O_2 TANK

First close the valve on the tank until the indicator on the meter drops to 0. Then allow any remaining oxygen to run out. (The water will stop bubbling and the liter gauge fall.) Then close the liter valve. Both of these turns are to the left.

RESPIRATOR

A respirator is a machine that forces air into the lungs and causes deep breathing. It is often referred to by trade name. Both the Bird respirator and the Bennet respirator are widely used, and reference to a "Bird" or a "Bennet" specifies the manufacturer of a respirator. When both are available, check the trademark to identify each.

Use of a respirator is ordered by a doctor when a patient's own breathing becomes impaired. Only someone trained in its use should operate a respirator.

A respirator is used for the following reasons:

       to help stretch and improve tone of respiratory muscles and lung tissues

       to help the patient cough up secretions without tiring

       to help deliver medication to deep areas of the lungs

       to help with the respirations of a patient with limited breathing ability

       to cause respirations in a patient who is completely unable to breathe by himself

The respirator can be used in two ways: (1) the patient or an attendant can have control and can start and stop the machine as desired or (2) the machine can be set on automatic control.

Respirator air is delivered to the patient by means of either a mouthpiece or a mask. Whichever method is used, it is very important that no air leaks around the mouthpiece or mask.

If a mouthpiece is used, the patient is told to bite on it gently and to close his lips tightly around it; he should not breathe through his nose while the respirator is in use. Sometimes a nasal clamp is used to prevent breathing through the nose.

If a mask is used, the patient's face should be wiped free of skin oil or sweat before the mask is applied. This helps to prevent the mask from slipping.

After starting the respirator, check all tube connections and the mouthpiece or mask for air leaks.

During use of the respirator, both the patient and the machine should be checked constantly. The patient should be checked for skin color changes, respiratory difficulty, and pulse change.

Until a patient becomes accustomed to a respirator, he may be frightened by it. If he is alert, he must be reassured. The operation of the machine should be explained to him, and he should control it whenever possible.

After he has become accustomed to it, he may become dependent on the machine and not make an effort to breathe. He may panic if the respirator is taken away. This patient also requires encouragement to breathe on his own. He may feel reassured if the respirator is left by his bedside, ready for use if necessary.

STEAM INHALATION

The doctor may order steam inhalations for the patient with respiratory infection or disease. Breathing moist hot air often helps relieve lung congestion. Sometimes medicine is given through steam inhalation.

Giving a Steam Inhalation

YOU NEED

    an electric vaporizer

    medication (if ordered by the doctor)

    2 bath towels

    water for vaporizer

    sputum cup

    tissues

YOU DO THIS

Be sure you understand how the particular vaporizer operates. If in doubt read the instructions or ask someone who knows.

Fill the vaporizer water container to the level marked.

If medicine has been ordered, put the correct amount in the vaporizer medicine container.

Take the vaporizer to the bedside and position it near to and directed toward the patient. Be sure to put the vaporizer where it cannot be a safety hazard. It can be placed on the floor or on a table.

Plug in and turn on the vaporizer and wait until it begins to steam.

Cover the patient's head and hair with one towel. Put the other around his shoulders. The towels absorb some of the moisture.

A croup tent can be made by draping a bathblanket over two I.V. poles positioned one on either side of the patient's head. A croup tent holds steam and so increases the concentration of vapor inhaled by the patient.

ARTIFICIAL RESPIRATION

Artificial respiration is the forcing of the breathing process after breathing has stopped.

Mouth-to-mouth resuscitation is the form of artificial respiration that is most effective for emergency use. When properly given, it can save the life of a person whose heart is beating but whose breathing has stopped.

Breathing may stop from many causes such as drowning, electric shock, poisoning, chest injury, and suffocation. The absence of the rise and fall of the chest is a good indication that breathing has stopped. Whether or not you know the cause of respiratory failure, begin mouth-to-mouth resuscitation.

Artificial respiration must be started within minutes after breathing stops, otherwise death cannot be prevented. A doctor or emergency service should be called as soon as possible. If you must choose between calling the doctor and giving resuscitation, choose to give resuscitation.

Giving Mouth-To-Mouth Resuscitation

YOU DO THIS

Position the patient flat on his back.

Reach into his mouth and throat with your fingers and remove anything that might be clogging the passage.

Using both of your hands, tilt the patient's head back so that the jaw juts out (lift his chin with one hand: press his forehead with your other palm).

Maintaining jutting jaw position, cover and seal the patient's open mouth with your mouth. Place your thumb and index finger at the end of the patient's nose.

Blow into the patient's mouth while pinching his nostrils shut.

Lift your mouth from the patient's and unclamp his nose. Take a breath and at the same time, press your other palm against the upper center of his abdomen.

Repeat about twenty times.

If you feel reluctant to place your mouth directly on the patient's, spread a handkerchief or other thin cloth over the patient's mouth before applying your own.

Part III

Special Conditions of Your Geriatric Patient

16

CARING FOR THE GERIATRIC PATIENT WHO HAS HAD A STROKE

STUDY GUIDE

What is a cerebral vascular accident?

What are some causes of CVA?

What are some symptoms of an approaching stroke?

What may happen to a person when stroke occurs?

Hemiplegia

What is hemiplegia?

If a CVA occurs on the left side of the brain, which side of the body is affected?

What are the effects of the bending muscles on the affected side of a patient with hemiplegia?

What are the three stages of hemiplegia?

Do all patients experience the three stages?

Nursing Care Plan

Tell 12 things that make up the nursing care plan of a patient with a CVA.

Tell how to arrange the unit of a patient whose left side is affected.

Vital Signs

How frequently are vital signs taken after a CVA?

When is a patient allowed out of bed?

Stroke Positioning

Give three reasons why stroke positioning and range-of-motion (R.O.M.) exercises are so important.

Give seven general rules for stroke positioning.

Tell how to position a patient on his back.

Tell how to position a patient on his side.

Tell how to position a patient on his abdomen.

Tell how to position a patient in a chair.

Rehabilitation Through A.D.L.

Tell how a patient can move himself from one side of the bed to the other.

Tell how a patient can roll himself over.

Tell how a patient can sit up by himself.

Tell how he can position himself with his legs dangling.

R.O.M. Exercises

What types of R.O.M. exercises are ordered for the patient with hemiplegia?

Skin Care

Why is it important to give the stroke patient frequent skin care?

Bowel and Bladder Control

What bowel and bladder care might the patient with a CVA need?

Bathing and Grooming

Which is better for a hemiplegia patient, a bath or a shower?

How can you shower a patient in the bathtub?

What aids can help the patient to bathe himself?

What type of razor is best for the stroke patient?

How can a stroke patient file the nails on his good hand?

Dressing the Hemiplegic Patient

What type of clothing should the patient wear?

What must you do for the forgetful patient?

Which side is always dressed first?

Which side is always undressed first?

In what positions can the patient be dressed?

What aids for shoes make it easier to put on and wear them?

Food and Fluid

What type of diet does the stroke patient usually receive?

What aids can help the patient with self-feeding?

When giving a plate of food to a patient, what should you do?

Communicating with the Patient

What happens to the patient's ability to communicate?

How can you establish a simple way to communicate with the patient?

What is aphasia?

Give some general rules to follow with the patient who has difficulty speaking?

Adaptive Equipment

What adaptive equipment might a stroke patient require?

AGE increases the chances of a person having a stroke or cerebral vascular accident (CVA). The word *cerebral* refers to the brain and the word *vascular* refers to the blood vessel system. Cerebral vascular accident therefore means an accident to the blood vessel system of the brain.

Normal nerve cells receive and interpret the messages of the senses (sight, hearing, smell, touch, and taste). Normal nerve cells also control movements. A CVA interferes with the blood supply to a part of the brain and, consequently, with the function of the nerve cells centered there.

CAUSES OF A CVA

Some of the many causes of a CVA are:
- a clot formed in a blood vessel of the brain.
- a clot formed elsewhere in the body but carried by the blood to the brain.
- a torn blood vessel that allows bleeding into the brain.
- pressure on a blood vessel caused by a tumor or swelling.
- a spasm of a brain artery.

PRE-STROKE SYMPTOMS

Signs that can indicate approaching stroke are: severe headache, blurred vision, difficulty in speaking, dizziness or fainting, and numbness in a hand or a side of the face.

UNDERSTANDING THE STROKE PATIENT

Until stroke occurs, the patient has the full use of his body. With the onset of stroke, he loses consciousness, and when he recovers, he does not know what has happened to him. He is frustrated, frightened, and unaware of the existence of his affected side.

He may be unable to speak or to understand when someone speaks to him.

If approached, spoken to, or given directions by one standing on his affected side, he may not understand or respond.

He may have visual problems. For example, from a plate of food he may eat only that which lies within the visual range of his unaffected side.

He may have hemiplegia (be unable to move the arm and leg on the affected side.)

The blood circulation on the affected side may be impaired.

He may have loss of sensation on the affected side.

He may be very forgetful and unable to concentrate.

He may tire easily.

His behavior may be inconsistent.

His balance while sitting and standing may be poor.

He may be incontinent of urine or feces or both.

HEMIPLEGIA

A CVA often causes hemiplegia, or loss of ability to move and loss of feeling in one side of the body. The paralysis occurs on the opposite side of the brain from the affected part. For example, when a CVA occurs on the left side of the brain, the right side of the body is affected.

Under normal conditions, muscles that bend a body part are stronger than muscles that straighten a part. When stroke occurs, the muscles that straighten are weakened (Fig. 56). The result is that the muscles that bend then pull the affected side.

One may observe the following:

quadriplegis- loss ability to move completed body

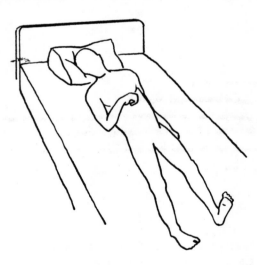

Figure 56. The differences between the affected side and the normal side of a hemiplegic patient. (From Elementary Rehabilitation Nursing Care, *U.S. Public Health Service, Division of Nursing.)*

The patient's head droops to the affected side.

The eyelid and mouth on the affected side may droop.

The arm is bent and hugs the chest.

Wrist, fingers, and thumb are bent.

SPECIAL CONDITIONS OF YOUR GERIATRIC PATIENT

The entire leg is extended and rotated outward.
The foot is on tiptoe and turned inward.
The entire body trunk tends to bend forward.

Stages of Hemiplegia

In the treatment of stroke, three progressive stages are recognized. Not all patients experience all three stages, however. Some may remain in the first stage; some progress to only the second stage. These stages are:

flaccid — the affected side is flaccid (weak and limp)
spastic — the affected side is spastic (develops tense muscles)
recovery — the affected side returns to usefulness and is neither flaccid nor spastic.

OVERALL NURSING CARE PLAN

Arrangement of patient's unit with consideration for the side affected
Vital signs (as ordered)
Stroke positioning
Turning and repositioning every two hours
Range-of-motion (R.O.M.) exercises (as ordered)
Skin care
Bowel and bladder control (as ordered)
Bathing and grooming
Food and fluid (as ordered and tolerated)
Communication with patient
Rehabilitation through activities of daily living
Adaptive equipment

SETTING UP A UNIT FOR THE STROKE PATIENT

Arrange the unit furniture so that the patient's unaffected side is toward the bedside stand and open unit area.

See that the bed
is a single or twin size
is waist high
has a firm mattress
has a bedboard
has a covered footboard
has a supply of towels, pillows, and blankets for positioning
has side rails

See that the bedside stand has the following:
a washbasin
soap in a soap dish
washcloths and towels
bedpan (and urinal if patient is male)
emesis basin
massage lotion

box of tissues
water pitcher
plastic water glass
bent paper straws or drinking tube

VITAL SIGNS

Blood pressure and temperature are taken often during the acute phase of a CVA. (The frequency depends on the doctor's instructions and the severity of the CVA.) The blood pressure readings are usually very unstable at first. The patient is kept on complete bed rest until the blood pressure stabilizes. It is not unusual for a stroke patient to have a fever during the acute signs of CVA.

STROKE POSITIONING

(*See* Chap. 10, "Your Geriatric Patient Needs Sleep, Rest, Positioning, and Transferring.")
Stroke positioning and R.O.M. exercises are extremely important in the care of a patient with a CVA because they prevent wasting (atrophy) of muscles and further crippling of the affected side. They also enable the patient to recover maximal function.

General Rules for Stroke Positioning

Place the patient on a firm mattress.
Don't elevate the head or foot of the bed.
Always keep the head and spine in alignment.
Do not position the patient on his affected side.
Alternate limb positions between extension and flexion.
Always keep the feet in neutral position.
Change the patient's position from back to good side, front, and then back every two hours.

Backlying (Supine) Position (Fig. 57)

See that the spine and head are in a straight line.
Do not use a pillow under the head.
Roll towels and fit them into the spaces under the neck, at the small of the back, under the knees, and in the affected hand (Fig. 58).
Place the soles of the feet flat against an upright brace in neutral position so that the feet cannot drop forward. Use a footboard or covered box as the brace.
Use a rolled blanket (trochanter roll), sandbags, or unopened food cans rolled in towels to brace the outside of the affected leg.

Side Position (Fig. 57)

Never turn the patient onto his affected side except for a few minutes, such as when making the bed.
Before turning the patient, always position the arm on the side to which the patient will turn. Raise that forearm beside the patient's head by rotating the shoulder. Cross the other arm over the chest.
After turning the patient, see that the spine and head are in a straight line.

SPECIAL CONDITIONS OF YOUR GERIATRIC PATIENT

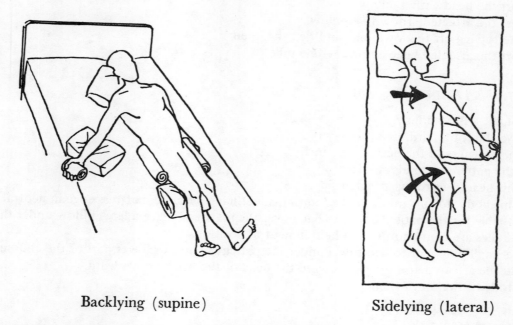

Backlying (supine)   Sidelying (lateral)

Figure 57. Backlying and sidelying positions for stroke patients. (From Elementary Rehabilitation Nursing Care, *U.S. Public Health Service, Division of Nursing.)*

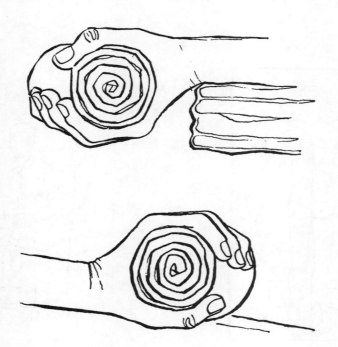

Figure 58. Positioning the affected hand of a stroke patient. (From Elementary Rehabilitation Nursing Care, *U.S. Public Health Service, Division of Nursing.)*

Support the head with a pillow.
Support the affected arm with a pillow.
Lift the top leg off the lower one and flex the knee.
Support the affected knee and leg with a pillow.

Frontlying (Prone) Position (Fig. 59)

Do not use a head pillow.
Remove the footboard.
Pull the mattress to the head of the bed.
Turn the patient onto his stomach.
Turn his head toward his affected side.
Move his body downward in the bed until his feet hang over the mattress edge in neutral position.
If it is impossible for the patient's feet to hang over the mattress, place a large pillow under the shins
so that the knees are bent and the feet held in neutral position.
Place a small pillow or folded towel under the patient's chest or lower part of the abdomen and hips.
Extend the affected arm upward toward the head of the bed or downward.
Put a rolled towel in the hand.

Chair Positioning (Fig. 59)

Use a chair with armrests.
After seating the patient, pull his buttocks forward a few inches. This allows him better seating
balance.

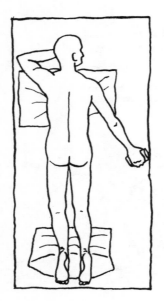

Facelying (prone)

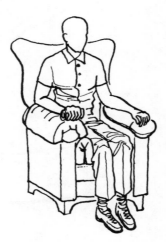

Sitting

Figure 59. Facelying and sitting positions for stroke patients. (From Elementary Rehabilitation Nursing Care, *U. S. Public Health Service, Division of Nursing.)*

SPECIAL CONDITIONS OF YOUR GERIATRIC PATIENT

See that his body is in good alignment.

Stabilize his affected leg by wedging a pillow or rolled towel between his thigh and the arm of the chair. Support the affected forearm with a pillow so that the shoulders are even.

Put a roll in the patient's hand.

Encourage the patient to hold his head erect and tilted to the unaffected side.

REHABILITATION THROUGH ACTIVITIES OF DAILY LIVING TRAINING (A.D.L.)

(*See* Chap. 5, "Your Geriatric Patient Needs Physical Therapy.")

A.D.L. training plays a very large part in the nursing care plan of the stroke patient. Many months of slow, continuous teamwork with the patient by the personnel of Physical Therapy, A.D.L. Training, and Nursing departments may be required in order to rehabilitate a stroke patient. Such work is often difficult but the satisfaction of watching a stroke patient respond to care is among the most rewarding experiences in nursing.

Self-Help Moving, Turning, and Positioning by the Hemiplegic

Moving from One Side of the Bed to the Other

Lying on his back, the patient hooks his good foot under his affected knee and pulls the leg until the knee is bent and the affected foot rests flat on the mattress.

He then puts his unaffected leg in the same position and pushes on his good foot, lifting the hips and moving them in the desired direction.

He moves his head and shoulders by pushing or pulling on the side rail with his good hand.

Rolling Over

The patient elevates both knees in the same manner as when he moves from one side of the bed to the other.

With his good hand, he pushes both knees in the direction of turn and allows the knees to fall. This partly rolls his body.

He rolls the rest of his body by pushing or pulling on the side rail with his good hand.

Sitting Up in Bed (Using a Bedrope)

A rope attached to the center of the foot of the bed can be used by the hemiplegic. Pulling on it with his good hand, he raises himself from a lying to a sitting position in bed.

Moving to Dangling Position (Using a Bedrope)

The patient lies on his back in the center of the bed and uses his good hand to cross his affected arm over his abdomen.

He moves his legs to the side of the bed until his feet and ankles extend over the side.

He pulls on the bedrope with his good hand, raising himself to a sitting position. His legs automatically fall over the bedside (Fig. 60).

It is very important to remember during all moving procedures that the CVA patient's affected side is deadweight, which, if off balance, can cause rapid overbalancing and falls.

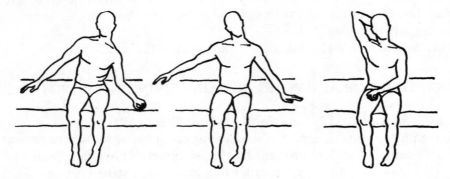

Figure 60. Stroke patient learning to balance in the dangling position. (From Elementary Rehabilitation Nursing Care, *U.S. Public Health Service, Division of Nursing.)*

R.O.M. EXERCISES

(*See* Chap. 5, "Your Geriatric Patient Needs Physical Therapy.")

Specific passive and active exercises are ordered at different stages of hemiplegia. As the patient progresses, he is taught to use his unaffected side to exercise his affected side (Figs. 61–63). You must be sure of which passive exercises you must do for the patient and which active exercises he should do by himself.

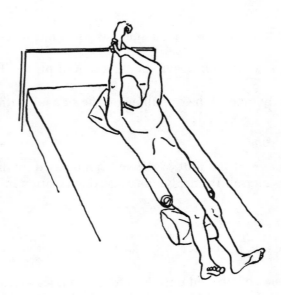

Figure 61. Stroke patient using good arm to exercise affected one. (From Elementary Rehabilitation Nursing Care, *U.S. Public Health Service, Division of Nursing.)*

SPECIAL CONDITIONS OF YOUR GERIATRIC PATIENT

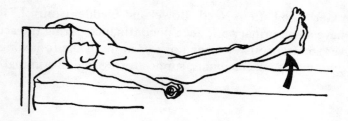

Figure 62.   Stroke patient using good leg to exercise affected one. (From Elementary Rehabilitation Nursing Care, *U.S. Public Health Service, Division of Nursing.)*

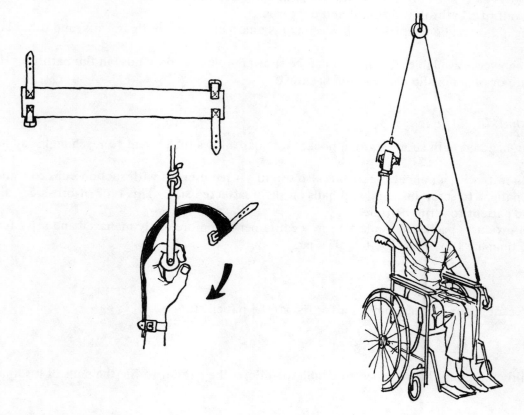

Figure 63.   A strap to secure handhold on an arm exerciser for a stroke patient.

SKIN CARE

(*See* Chap. 12, "Your Geriatric Patient Needs Skin Care.")

Because of changes in his blood circulation, incontinence, and dead weight of his paralyzed side, the patient with a CVA is susceptible to pressure sores. Skin care should be given at every opportunity.

BOWEL AND BLADDER CONTROL

(*See* Chap. 14, "Your Geriatric Patient Needs Bowel and Bladder Control.")

Most stroke patients have some urinary and fecal incontinence during the acute phase of illness. Any one patient may recover spontaneously or need one or more of the following: care for incontinence, Foley catheter drainage, condom drainage, enemas, suppositories, digital stimulation to remove feces, and retraining.

BATHING AND GROOMING

Bathing

The hemiplegic requires bed baths until he is allowed out of bed.

Once he is able to be up and about, he should have showers rather than baths, because transferring him in and out of a bathtub is difficult and dangerous.

During a shower, he will need help washing his unaffected arm, both armpits, and other areas he cannot reach.

If no shower is available, the patient can be showered with a spray hose in the bathtub. He should sit in the tub or on a nonslip chair with a backrest.

A.D.L. Bath Aids

A long-handled bath sponge with a pocket for soap allows the patient to reach and soap nearly all his body.

A bath mitt with a pocket for soap is also useful. A hand brush with suction cups to stabilize it allows the patient to scrub his hand and nails on the unaffected side. This type of brush can also be used by the patient to scrub dentures.

Toilet products packaged in plastic spray containers are more easily managed and safer for the hemiplegic than are those in screw top glass jars.

Shaving

An electric razor is easier and safer for the stroke patient to use.

Nail Care

A nailfile or emery board taped to a tabletop allows the patient to file the nails of his unaffected hand.

Dressing the Hemiplegic Patient

Clothing should be oversized, fit loosely, and have easy closures in front or at the side. Wrap-around or front-opening dresses with large buttons or Velcro fasteners are best. Short sleeves are easiest to manage. If sleeves are long, the wrist edges should be wide enough to admit the hand with ease. Halfslips are easier than full-slips for the female patient. Ready-tied bow ties are best for men. Button flies are easier for the patient to manage than zippers.

Forgetfulness often accompanies hemiplegia. The patient therefore may need step-by-step reminders in order to dress himself.

The affected side is always dressed first.

The unaffected side is always undressed first.

It is usually easiest to dress or undress the lower part of the body in bed.

If the patient has poor balance, the upper part of his body can be dressed while he is lying in bed by turning him from side to side.

If the patient has good balance, the upper part of his body can be dressed while he sits on the side of the bed.

Shoelaces must be tied securely. Elastic shoelaces are best because they do not need tying.

A long-handled shoehorn makes it easier for a patient to put on his shoes.

FOOD AND FLUID

(*See* Chap. 9, "Your Geriatric Patient Needs Food and Fluid Balance.")

The doctor usually orders a high protein diet to help rebuild the stroke patient's body. In the early acute stage, the patient may be on a liquid diet, with soft solids added as he is able to tolerate them. Later, he may receive a regular diet.

At the self-help stage of eating, the patient may need much encouragement because he may be very untidy and clumsy with eating utensils. A damp sponge-rubber mat under a dish will stabilize it. Nonbreakable dishware and drinking cup or glass, a spoon rather than a fork, and a rocker-handled knife may help him to feed himself better. One dish at a time is best at first.

It may be necessary when offering food to a hemiplegic to draw his attention to what is on the plate within the visual field of his affected side. He may be unaware of it and eat only the food he can see. Rotating his plate during the meal brings the food within his range of vision.

COMMUNICATING WITH THE PATIENT

After the onset of a stroke, the patient may be unable to speak and sometimes hard to understand. It is important to establish a simple way to communicate as soon as possible. This is best done by agreeing to signals and then asking simple questions requiring a yes or no answer. For example, tell the patient to raise his good hand if the answers to your questions are yes. Phrase questions simply.

Examples: "Are you hungry?"
"Are you cold?"
"Can you hear me?"

Aphasia

An aphasic patient is one with a speech problem. Aphasia is common in a stroke patient. It is important to understand that the aphasic patient has no memory of speech and must relearn to speak.

General Rules

Allow the patient as much freedom to speak as possible.
Let him make mistakes.
Give the patient opportunities to hear speech.
Speak to the patient in short, simple, clear sentences.
Speak slowly.
Encourage the patient to speak and praise his efforts.
Don't force the patient to speak or to see people if he doesn't want to do it.

Don't talk for the patient.

Don't interrupt while the patient tries to speak.

Don't insist that the patient speak perfectly.

Don't scold if he doesn't speak.

Never become angry. That increases the patient's difficulties.

Don't remind the patient that he could speak before he became ill.

Never isolate the patient.

Don't expect thanks for any attention that you show.

If the patient is doing something, don't interrupt, even though his activity may appear foolish to you.

Don't make unrealistic demands that the patient cannot possibly meet.

Don't allow the patient to be disturbed by unnecessary problems.

ADAPTIVE EQUIPMENT

(*See* Chap. 6, "Your Geriatric Patient Needs Adaptive Equipment.")

In the course of recovery, a stroke patient may require many pieces of adaptive equipment: a leg brace, special shoes, a wheelchair, an arm sling, a cane.

17

CARING FOR THE GERIATRIC PATIENT WITH ARTHRITIS

STUDY GUIDE

What is arthritis?

What parts of the body does it affect?

What happens to people with progressive arthritis?

What nursing care may such a patient require?

How can arthritis affect a patient's personality?

How should you behave with an arthritic patient?

Tell how to set up a unit for an arthritic patient.

Medication

What medication is often ordered for arthritis?

With what should the medication be given?

What effect may the medication have on the patient?

How should you deal with that effect?

Rest

What should an arthritic patient avoid?

How much rest should an arthritic patient have?

Positioning

Tell how an arthritic patient should be positioned in bed and in a chair.

Bathing

What type of bath is best for the arthritic patient? Why?

Name some bath aids that can help the arthritic patient.

Physical Therapy

What kinds of range of motion (R.O.M.) exercises may be ordered for the patient?

How many times should each be done?

What type of heat should be used on an arthritic patient?

Name some forms of moist heat therapy.

Tell what you need to prepare a paraffin bath.

What is the maximal temperature to which the paraffin should be heated? What temperature should the paraffin be before use by a patient?

What should you do with the paraffin on the patient's hands or feet when the treatment is over?

Tell how to prepare and give contrast baths.

What should be the temperatures of the basins of water?

Tell how to prepare and apply moist hot towels.

Food and Fluid

What should a good diet for arthritics accomplish?

Why is excess weight undesirable in an arthritic patient?

What eating peculiarities may the arthritic develop?

Why should close watch be kept of the arthritic's food intake?

What is your responsibility toward the patient with an eating device?

Bowel Control

How can you make it easier for the arthritic patient to have bowel movements?

Why should close watch be kept of his bowel movements?

Rehabilitation

How often may an arthritic patient need rehabilitation?

What should you do if you notice a patient having difficulty with a specific A.D.L. device?

ARTHRITIS is a chronic disease that causes inflammation and pain in the joints. It can affect fingers, wrists, elbows, shoulders, the spinal vertebrae, hips, knees, ankles, and toes. The cause is unknown, although two types of arthritis are recognized: rheumatoid arthritis and osteoarthritis.

Most older people suffer periodic attacks of arthritis, but with some the disease is progressive. The patient experiences intense pain and joint changes that make movement difficult.

Such a patient may require a great deal of personal attention and nursing care. Because his movements are slow and painful, nursing care may take longer than with another patient. Then, too, the personality of the arthritic patient is often affected by the disease. He may be very emotional, depressed, complaining, and demanding.

His attitude, combined with his slowness, can be very irritating unless you remind yourself that he does not want to be the way he is. He cannot change. You must be always calm, patient, kind, and gentle. Try to imagine how his pain and frustration must feel. Remember how much he needs you.

OVERALL NURSING CARE PLAN

Set up unit for arthritic patient
Medication
Rest
Positioning
Bathing and grooming
Physical therapy
Adaptive equipment
Food and fluid
Bowel control
Rehabilitation through training in activities of daily living (A.D.L.)

SETTING UP A UNIT FOR THE ARTHRITIC PATIENT

Place the bed where it isn't near a window or other source of draft.
The unit should include the following:

an adjustable bed
a hinged bedboard to allow for elevating the head of the bed
a firm mattress covered with a foam mattress
a flat head pillow
a covered footboard
a comfortable armchair with raised seat level

MEDICATION

Arthritic patients often receive aspirin or a pain medicine containing it. Aspirin should be given with milk or other food. This medicine often causes sweating. The patient's clothing should be changed when sweating occurs, and care should be taken to avoid drafts.

REST

An important part of the care plan is sufficient rest. The patient should have a quiet, regular routine that includes as much occupational and recreational therapy as he enjoys. The patient should not become overtired, excited, or emotional, however.
Night bed rest should be 8–10 hours.
Daytime bed rest (two daily 1-hour periods) should be required.

POSITIONING

(*See* Chap. 10, "Your Geriatric Patient Needs Sleep, Rest, Positioning, and Transferring.")

In a Bed

Use a firm mattress.
See that spine and head are in a straight line.

Use a flat head pillow.

Position the joints in mild extension.

When moving the patient, do not take hold of joints.

Do not use pillows under the knees.

Use a footboard.

Do not allow bedding to touch the feet. Tuck the top bedding over and around the footboard. If necessary, use a bed cradle.

In a Chair

Use a comfortable chair with padded armrests and a raised seat. A thick foam cushion on a hard surface may be used to raise the level.

Position patient's body in alignment.

BATHING AND GROOMING

A daily 30-minute tub bath is better than a shower because soaking in hot water relieves pain and stiffness. Most patients prefer an early morning bath because it limbers them for the day's activities. When possible, however, the patient should select the time. Sometimes more than one daily bath is allowed.

Various aids, such as bath mitt, soap on a cotton rope necklace, long-handled plastic reaching tongs, and a rubber bath pillow for the head, are available. Thought should be given to the patient's specific limitations of motion and A.D.L. aids selected to meet them (Fig. 64). The A.D.L. nurse and physical therapist usually choose the equipment but welcome suggestions from patients and others, such as aides, who work closely with the patient. (*See* Chap. 5, "Your Geriatric Patient Needs Physical Therapy.") Skin lotion should be applied generously because long baths tend to dry the skin.

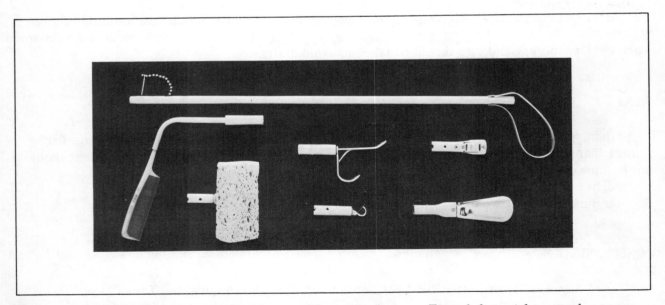

Figure 64. A reaching rod (at top) with interchangeable devices. From left to right: comb, sponge, reaching hook, grasping hook (below), magnet, and shoehorn (below). (Reprinted by permission of © J. A. Preston Corp., 1971.)

PHYSICAL THERAPY

Specific passive and active range of motion (R.O.M.) exercises may be ordered. Unless the doctor specifies the number, each exercise should be done no more than five times during one exercise period.

Heat is helpful in relieving pain and stiffness. Only moist heat, however, should be used. Methods of heat therapy often used include 30-minute tub baths in water at 105°F., hydrocollator pads, paraffin baths, contrast baths, and moist hot towels.

Paraffin Bath or Dip (for hands and feet)

YOU NEED

    2 oz. of mineral oil

    2 oz. of paraffin

    a bath thermometer

    double boiler large enough for the hand or foot to enter the top

---

YOU DO THIS

Put paraffin and mineral oil in top of double boiler.

Put bath thermometer in paraffin.

Put water in bottom of double boiler.

Put boiler top inside boiler bottom.

Heat over low flame until paraffin melts.

Watch bath thermometer. Do not let paraffin heat to more than 120°F. or it tends to burn.

Turn off heat.

Remove top of boiler.

Let paraffin cool to 110°F.

Dip patient's hands (or feet) repeatedly, one at a time, into and out of the melted paraffin until a thick film has formed on both hands (or feet).

After 30 minutes, pull the paraffin off and replace it in the boiler top to be used for the next treatment.

Most geriatric nursing homes use a commercial paraffin bath machine (Fig. 65).

---

specific passive and active range of motion (see chapter 19) exercises that can be carried out. Dulcet the doctor specifies the number of times each should be carried out, usually only once or twice during one exercise period.

Heat is helpful in relieving pain and stiffness. Only those heat treatments should be used, methods of heat therapy, often used in the geriatric tub baths, may be used. Heat therapy includes hot paraffin baths, contrast baths, and infra-red lamps.

Paraffin Bath or Dip for hand

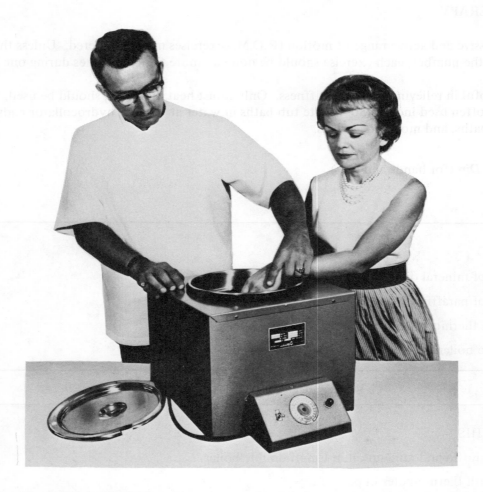

Figure 65. A paraffin bath. (Reprinted by permission of © J. A. Preston Corp., 1971.)

Contrast Bath (for hands and feet)

> YOU NEED
>> plastic cover for table
>> basin with water at 65°F.
>> basin with water at 105°F.
>> bath thermometer
>> towel

SPECIAL CONDITIONS OF YOUR GERIATRIC PATIENT

YOU DO THIS

Plunge hands (or feet) into basin of hot water for 4 minutes; then plunge them into basin of cold water for 1 minute.

Repeat for 20 minutes.

Moist Hot Towels

YOU NEED

2 or more small-sized turkish towels

large double boiler

bath thermometer

plastic square

1 dry bath towel

skin lotion

YOU DO THIS

Wet towels and wring dry.

Fold into small pads.

Put folded towels in the top part of the double boiler.

Put water in the bottom part of the double boiler.

Put top in bottom part of double boiler.

Heat until towels are 110°F. (no hotter).

Take double boiler to bedside.

Prepare patient.

Remove one moist towel and apply.

Cover with plastic square.

Cover plastic with dry towel.

Remove after 10 minutes and apply other moist towel in the same way.

ADAPTIVE EQUIPMENT

The arthritic patient often requires walking aids: special shoes, cane or Loftstrand crutch, a walker. When the disease is severe and deforming, he may need a wheelchair. However, every effort should be made to keep him as mobile as possible and to prevent permanent stiffness of joints. The disease has acute periods during which one or more joints become more intensely inflamed. When these periods occur, the doctor may order a temporary rest for the joint. For example, an arm sling may be ordered to rest the arm and shoulder until the acute stage passes.

FOOD AND FLUID

A good diet for an arthritic furnishes all the essentials for proper nourishment but keeps the patient's weight at a minimum. Excess weight aggravates arthritis. Since weight is an individual condition, and geriatric arthritics often require other dietary specifications, the doctor orders a diet to suit the patient. (*Example:* An overweight arthritic patient may have high blood pressure and diabetes. In that case, the doctor would order a low-calorie, salt-free and sugar-free diet.)

The arthritic patient often needs encouragement to eat. If eating involves pain, the patient tends to eat less and to select food from his meal. He may also reject or pick at food when emotional. By doing so, he may change the nutritional balance of his diet. Close watch should be taken of the patient's eating pattern, and you should report changes in the patient's food intake to the charge nurse or doctor.

Many A.D.L. aids are available to help the patient with arthritis involving the arm and hand. The physical therapist and A.D.L. nurse usually work with the patient to discover which A.D.L. aids are best for the individual. Your responsibility is to see that the patient uses the prescribed feeding aid. Although it may appear easier for you to feed this patient, you would be doing him harm by doing so, if a feeding device has been ordered.

BOWEL CONTROL

Sitting on the toilet, commode, or bedpan often involves pain for this patient, and he may tend to put off bowel movements until fecal impaction occurs. Every effort should be made to make the patient as comfortable as possible while he has a bowel movement. A raised toilet seat (Fig. 66) and correct bedpan positioning are two of the many ways by which bowel movements can be made easier.

Close watch should be kept on the patient's bowel movements and changes reported to the charge nurse. The doctor usually orders laxatives and enemas as needed to keep the bowels in good working condition.

REHABILITATION THROUGH A.D.L. TRAINING

There is a limit to how much a patient with progressive arthritis can be rehabilitated. He may also require periodic rehabilitation to meet his decreasing abilities with different devices. He should be kept as self-sufficient as possible, however, and encouraged in self-care. Changes in his ability to use A.D.L. devices and to perform daily activities should be reported to the charge nurse or doctor.

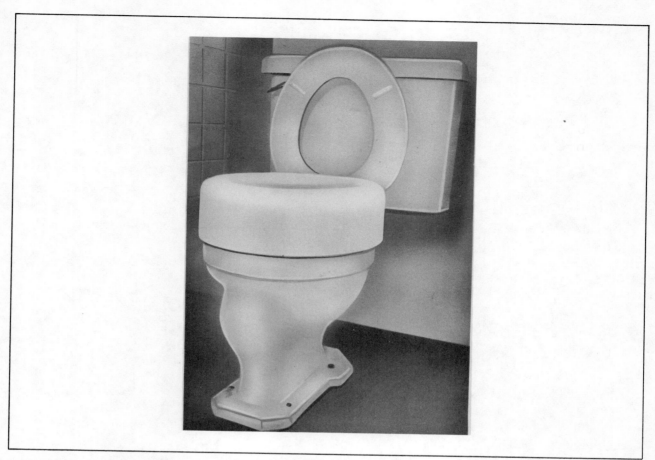

Figure 66.   A raised toilet seat. (Reprinted by permission of © J. A. Preston Corp., 1971.)

18

CARING FOR THE GERIATRIC PATIENT WITH A MENTAL DISORDER

STUDY GUIDE

What are some aspects of a patient's life that influence a mental disorder?

What are the two main causes of mental disorders?

What are some conditions that can trigger a mental disorder of emotional origin?

What have scientists discovered about isolation?

To what do disorders from an emotional cause respond?

What are some physical causes of mental disorders at all ages of human life?

What two types due to physical causes occur only in older people?

Can a person with chronic brain disease be cured?

What happens to the brain of a person with chronic brain disease?

Can a patient have more than one form of mental disorder?

Why do patients with chronic brain disease need special care?

What are some symptoms of mental disorders?

What are your special duties as an aide toward the geriatric patient with a mental disorder?

Give the seven rules to be observed when a patient with a mental disorder has a visitor.

What special care should be taken during treatments?

How would you take the temperature of a disturbed person?

What is gavage?

REGARDLESS of cause, a mental disorder is always complex and peculiar to the individual because it includes all his life experiences, health and family histories, and social and economic backgrounds. The main cause of a mental disorder, however, is always either emotional or physical.

EMOTIONAL CAUSES OF MENTAL DISORDERS

Mental disorders of emotional origin are very common among geriatric patients and are often combined with physical causes. Loneliness, fears of the future, of death, of rejection by children, and frustrations over failing vision, hearing, or mobility can trigger mental disorder in a geriatric patient.

Of all these, perhaps loneliness is the worst. Scientists working with healthy animals produce mental disorders in them simply by isolating them from others of their kind. When isolation is added to the physical disabilities of human aging, it is easy to imagine the unfortunate effect.

Mental disorders from emotional causes often respond very favorably if the patient receives loving, protective care and stimulating society.

PHYSICAL CAUSES OF MENTAL DISORDERS

Many mental disorders of physical cause can affect both young and old. Some of these causes are infections, drugs, alcohol, head injury, brain tumor, and inadequate diet.

Two other disorders of physical cause occur only in older people. They are hardening of the head arteries (cerebral arteriosclerosis) and death of brain tissue from age (senile brain disease). These two diseases cause destruction of brain cells and are known as chronic brain disease.

Once destroyed, brain cells cannot be restored. Brain damage is permanent, and a person can never learn, understand, remember, or manage a body function if the brain control center has been destroyed. If the speech area is destroyed, for example, the patient cannot speak words unless another area of his brain is trained to accept the function. Then he must relearn to speak, just as a child. He has no knowledge or memory of speech to help him.

Some older people have both forms of chronic brain disease. Although these patients should be maintained at the highest level of mental ability possible, they need special care as they become less and less able to function. Most eventually become irrational and incontinent, and require total care. Because they are distressing to other geriatric patients, those with advanced chronic brain disease are usually kept apart from other levels of geriatric nursing home care.

SYMPTOMS OF MENTAL DISORDERS

Whether originating from emotional or physical causes, all mental disorders cause changes in the personality of a person. Some signs of such changes include the following:

anxiety
confusion
depression
overactivity
underactivity
talkativeness
silence
angry outbursts
incontinence
weeping without cause
laughing without cause
talking to one's self

SPECIAL CONDITIONS OF YOUR GERIATRIC PATIENT

withdrawal from others
complaining or demanding behavior
forgetfulness

YOUR DUTIES AS A GERIATRIC AIDE

Observe the patient's physical and mental conditions and report changes.

See that the patient has food, water, and bowel and bladder control.

Do not react to the patient's actions. If the patient has an angry outburst, for example, do not become angry or scold him. Keep calm and be kind at all times.

Always talk to the patient when you are with him.

Touch the patient in a slow, gentle way whenever possible. Touch is especially important for patients with loss of hearing or vision.

Use resocialization and remotivation techniques regardless of whether the patient appears to respond. (*See* Chap. 7, "Your Geriatric Patient Needs Remotivation and Resocialization.")

Never tease, bully, laugh at, or talk about a patient in his presence.

Keep the patient clean, neat, and dressed in attractive clothes.

Set standards for the patient who is able to meet them. (*Example:* "Zip up your trousers. All the men here keep their trousers zippered.")

Put the patient in social situations that he can tolerate. (*Examples:* feed him with others; let him sit in a group to watch television; or put his wheelchair near a busy doorway.) Observe his reactions to these situations.

Find out whether the patient receives medication for his mental condition and how that medication can affect him.

VISITORS

A patient is cleaned, dressed neatly, quieted, and prepared for a visitor.

No information should be given to a visitor about the patient, his treatment, or the nursing facility by anyone except the doctor or charge nurse.

Visitors should obtain special permission to bring gifts to patients. Any gift should be examined to prevent the patient from receiving something harmful.

No patient should sign papers during a visit.

No patient or visitor should smoke or have matches.

If the patient appears to be disturbed by the visit, the visitor should be asked to leave.

Unusual behavior by the patient or the visitor should be reported to the charge nurse.

SPECIAL CARE WITH TREATMENTS

Special care must be taken to prevent the patient from misinterpreting a treatment. He should be approached in a gentle way and the treatment explained to him before it is started.

Treatments are usually given by two persons, especially when the genital area is involved.

As little equipment as necessary is used in order to lessen the patient's alarm. Any equipment is made of unbreakable material, when possible, and kept out of the patient's reach.

Procedures are done quickly.

Taking Temperatures

Rectal temperatures are taken on disturbed patients. The attendant remains with the patient and holds the thermometer while it is inserted. Disturbed patients are apt to bite mouth thermometers.

Medicines

Paper cups, spoons, and straws are used to give medicines.

A person giving medicine should stay with a patient until the dose is swallowed. It is often necessary to check the inside of the mouth to determine that a pill is swallowed. Most disturbed patients are treated with drugs that help them to adjust to life. It is most important that they take these drugs in the right dosage and at the right times.

Gavage

This is a method of feeding used when a patient refuses to eat. A tube is passed through the nose and into the stomach. The tube is called a gavage, Levin, or gastric tube. Eggnogs, juices, formulas, and medicines may be given in this way, if so ordered.

HOME CARE

In caring for a disturbed person at home, the basic rules and philosophy used in institutional care should be applied. Never leave the patient alone. Prevent him from injuring himself or others. See that he receives adequate physical care. Treat him with kindness and understanding. Do not let him be aware of your problems, frustrations, or disappointments. Create a safe, calm place for him to live.

SPECIAL CONDITIONS OF YOUR GERIATRIC PATIENT

19

CARING FOR THE GERIATRIC DIABETIC PATIENT

STUDY GUIDE

What is diabetes?

How is it controlled?

Why is diabetes dangerous for the geriatric patient?

Tell how to test for sugar in the urine with Clinitest.

Tell how to test for acetone in the urine with Acetest.

Tell how to test for sugar in the urine with Testape.

Who orders the special diet for a diabetic patient?

Give seven specific sources of sugar that are forbidden to a diabetic patient.

What can be used as a sugar substitute?

Why must insulin be given?

By what ways is insulin given?

What are symptoms of insulin shock? Of diabetic coma?

Why should a diabetic patient have regular eye examinations?

Why is positioning important?

Why is skin care especially important?

Tell some special means of skin care for the diabetic geriatric patient.

Who should trim the toenails of a diabetic patient?

What is an amputation?

What is gangrene?

What general rules should you follow when caring for a patient with an amputation? _sugar-False_

DIABETES is a disease resulting from the body's inability to make enough insulin, a glandular secretion that controls the body's ability to utilize sugar. Insulin is produced in the pancreas. Without sufficient insulin, too much sugar stays in the blood and spills over into the urine.

To correct this imbalance the person's diet must be controlled to limit sugar intake, and in most instances insulin must be given. Insulin may be administered by injection or orally. The amount of insulin must balance the amounts and kinds of food the patient eats.

The doctor orders the following special care:

   urine tests for sugar and acetone at exact times
   a special diet
   insulin to be given in exact doses at exact times
   skin care

SPECIAL CONSIDERATIONS IN GERIATRICS

Reports on blood tests for detection of diabetes should be part of every evaluation and reevaluation of a geriatric patient. Many patients develop the disease in later life, although such cases are often mild and can be controlled by diet alone or by diet and daily oral medication.

Diabetes can be very dangerous for the geriatric patient, however. Not only is he subject to the problems of the disease, but diabetes also complicates many other common diseases of aging. The diabetic patient with varicose veins who develops varicose ulcers, for example, is less likely to respond to treatment than is the nondiabetic patient. Diabetes increases susceptibility to any infection and lengthens any healing process in the patient. Gangrene and the necessity for amputation can develop from a pin scratch or any improperly trimmed toenail. Diabetes can cause permanent loss of eyesight.

URINE TESTING IS VERY IMPORTANT

A Clinitest or Testape urine testing package can be purchased at any drugstore.

Keep testing equipment together on a tray. Post the Clinitest or Testape chart on a nearby wall or inside a medicine cabinet door.

How to Test for Sugar with Clinitest

YOU DO THIS

Collect a fresh specimen from the patient at each of the times the doctor has ordered.

Take urine to the utility room.

Use a medicine dropper to drop 5 drops of urine into a test tube.

Rinse the dropper and drop 10 drops of water into the same test tube.

Drop 1 test tablet of Clinitest into the test tube. Do not handle test tablets. (Pour 1 tablet into the bottle cap and then into test tube.)

Watch the reaction until 15 seconds after the reaction stops.

Shake the test tube gently.

Hold the test tube near the Clinitest chart and compare the colors.

If the result is negative, mark this on a record sheet and give the reading to the charge nurse.

If the result is positive, mark the exact reading on a record sheet and report the reading to the charge nurse or doctor at once.

How to Test for Acetone with Acetest

YOU DO THIS

Put an Acetest tablet on a dry white paper.

Use a medicine dropper to drop 1 or 2 drops of urine on the tablet.

Wait 60 seconds and compare the color of the tablet with the Acetest color chart.

Mark the exact reading on the record sheet and report the reading to the charge nurse.

How to Test for Sugar with Testape

Another means of testing urine for sugar is with Testape. It is simple to use and is packaged in a small plastic container that is convenient to carry.

YOU DO THIS

Collect urine in clean container.

Check the expiration date on the Testape container. Do not use tape with an expired date.

See that your hands are clean and dry.

Lift the top lid of the container. Pull out about one and one-half inches of tape. Continue to hold tape straight out while closing lid. After closing lid, jerk tape to release it from container.

Pinch one end of the tape between your thumb and forefinger and quickly dip the other end into the urine; remove tape immediately.

Continue to hold tape for one minute to allow for complete color development.

Match tape color against color chart on Testape container.

If tape color reads +++, wait an additional one-half minute (30 seconds) to see if there are further color changes. Compare tape color and color chart again.

Write down and report results of the test.

If the tests for sugar and acetone are strongly positive, the doctor may order extra insulin to be given before the next meal. He may change the patient's diet.

DIET IS VERY IMPORTANT

The doctor provides the patient with a special diet and instructs the patient on using it. The patient is allowed to select, from specific listings of foods and exact portions, the menu for each of his meals. Only those foods and portions are permitted. *The patient must not eat other foods or amounts.* No sugars are allowed:

No sugar for table or tray use
No sugar-sweetened canned fruit
No sugar-sweetened gelatins, puddings, or ice creams
No sugar-sweetened pies, cakes, cookies, or candy
No sugar-sweetened soft drinks
No alcoholic drinks (Alcohol has a high sugar content.)
No oranges or other very sweet fruits unless specifically ordered

Saccharin may be used as a sugar substitute.

The patient must eat all the food prepared for his meal. If everything is not eaten, a description of what he left must be reported. (*Example:* The patient refused his entire serving of meat. He ate his vegetables and fruit but left half his bread and butter.) A substitute meal may be necessary to balance his food intake with his insulin intake.

INSULIN IS VERY IMPORTANT

It must be given exactly as ordered, to balance the patient's intake of food.
Insulin for injection must be kept in the refrigerator.
Oral insulin need not be kept in the refrigerator.
The patient must be watched for symptoms of:

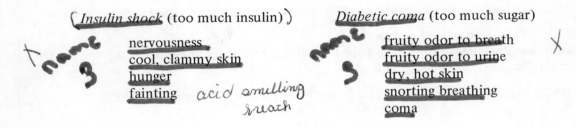

(*Insulin shock* (too much insulin))

nervousness
cool, clammy skin
hunger
fainting   *acid smelling breath*

Diabetic coma (too much sugar)

fruity odor to breath
fruity odor to urine
dry, hot skin
snorting breathing
coma

If these symptoms appear, a doctor must be called at once.

The diabetic patient who goes alone from his home should wear an identification bracelet or carry a card which states, "I am a Diabetic." Then, in the event of coma or shock, correct treatment can be given at once.

EYE EXAMINATIONS BY A DOCTOR WHO SPECIALIZES IN EYE CONDITIONS ARE VERY IMPORTANT

The diabetic should have his eyes examined every six months. Proper and prompt treatment can prevent or delay blindness.

POSITIONING IS VERY IMPORTANT

The geriatric diabetic patient is more prone to decubitis ulcers, and if one develops, it is less likely to heal than in a nondiabetic patient. This patient, therefore, should have frequent checks on body alignment, activity, and skin condition. He should change position frequently.

SKIN CARE IS VERY IMPORTANT

Every diabetic should have a routine of skin inspection and care that eliminates the possibility of infection from cuts, scratches, or pressure sores.

His fingernails and toenails should be trimmed by a doctor, podiatrist, or other specially trained person. Hangnails should not be allowed to develop.

He should never wear clothing that binds, cuts, scratches, or irritates the skin. He should never wear shoes that pinch or rub.

He should use a soft toothbrush, use mouthwash frequently.

DIABETIC AMPUTATION

Amputation means surgical removal of a part of the body, such as a finger, arm, foot, or leg. With advancing age, blood circulation in the feet and legs becomes less and less efficient. As a result, infections there take longer to heal. When diabetes is also present, an infection can quickly spread through the foot or leg until gangrene develops. (Gangrene is the death of tissue from infection and inadequate blood circulation.) When this occurs, the affected part must be amputated to prevent the gangrene from spreading.

General Rules for Care of a Patient with an Amputation

(*See* Chap. 6, "Your Geriatric Patient Needs Adaptive Equipment.")

Make frequent checks on the amputee to be sure that, whether he is lying, sitting, or standing, his body is in good alignment so that his blood flows freely to all parts.

When the patient is in bed:

See that he does not lie with flexed knees or curved spine.
See that no pillow is placed under the hip or knee of the amputed leg.

See that no pillow is placed between the patient's thighs.
See that the stump never hangs over the side of the bed.
See that the patient does not spread his legs wide.

When the patient is standing with crutches:

See that he uses the crutches correctly.
Never allow him to rest the stump on a crutch handle.

When the patient is using a wheelchair:

Keep the stump elevated in line with the hip; never let it hang over the seat.

SPECIAL CONDITIONS OF YOUR GERIATRIC PATIENT

20

CARING FOR THE GERIATRIC CARDIAC AND RESPIRATORY PATIENT

STUDY GUIDE

How does aging affect the heart and blood vessels?

What are five common forms of heart disease in the aged?

What is an E.K.G. or E.C.G.?

What does it show?

Name acute symptoms of heart trouble.

What is a coronary care unit?

What is a cardiac monitor?

Tell ways in which to assure the patient of physical rest.

How is mental rest assured?

How is emotional rest assured?

How is a cardiac patient positioned in bed?

If a sign on a cardiac patient's bed reads, "Keep Head of Bed Elevated," should you lower the bed to change the linen?

What rules must you follow when a patient is receiving oxygen?

What types of special diets may a doctor order for a heart patient?

Tell 15 ways a low-salt diet should be followed.

Tell ten ways in which a low-cholesterol diet should be followed.

Tell seven ways in which a low-calorie diet should be followed.

What are some symptoms of a patient with chronic heart disease?

Give six general rules for care of a patient with chronic heart disease.

What can you expect when a patient is taking diuretic medication?

What should you do for the patient who is taking nitroglycerine?

What should you do when the patient is allowed to control his oxygen tank?

What three respiratory diseases are common in geriatric patients?

How do colds, flus, and pneumonia affect patients with respiratory diseases?

What should you give a person with a productive cough?

What physical things do you notice about respiratory patients?

What bed position is most comfortable for respiratory patients?

How does postural drainage benefit a patient with respiratory disease?

What do you need in order to give postural drainage when using an upholstered arm chair?

Tell how to give postural drainage to a patient by using a low-backed upholstered arm chair.

Tell how to collect a sputum specimen.

CARDIOVASCULAR, OR HEART AND BLOOD VESSEL SYSTEM

The heart is a muscular organ. Blood, filled with carbon dioxide and other wastes from all the cells of the body, enters the heart from the system of veins.

Contractions of the heart muscle send this blood to the lungs to be purified of carbon dioxide and wastes, and to take in oxygen.

The oxygenated blood returns to the heart and is pumped through the system of arteries to feed and give oxygen to all cells of the body.

RESPIRATORY SYSTEM

Air, breathed in through the nose and mouth, passes along the trachea, or windpipe, past the larynx, or voice box, into the bronchial tubes, or main air tubes of the lungs. Many smaller tubes branch off the bronchial tubes and those tubes branch until much of the lung is filled with tiny air passages. Most of the remaining lung is filled with tiny blood vessels.

Fresh air, containing oxygen, is inhaled into the lungs and exchanged for one of the body's waste products, carbon dioxide, which is exhaled. The carbon dioxide is carried by the blood system to the lungs from all body cells.

The act of breathing is controlled by a large muscle that lies under the lungs. This muscle is the diaphragm. The expansion of the diaphragm causes a sucking in of air, or inhalation. The contraction of the diaphragm squeezes air from the lungs. This is called exhalation.

Inhalation is also called inspiration.

Exhalation is also called expiration.

One act of inspiration and expiration is called respiration

Because the heart and lungs are connected and dependent on each other, disease of one usually causes distress in the other.

Aging causes changes in the heart and blood vessels that result in disease. Most geriatric patients eventually suffer from some chronic form of this disease. Some common forms of heart and blood vessel disease are:

Know {
    hypertension or high blood pressure
    arteriosclerosis or hardening of the arteries
    coronary thrombosis or heart attack
    aneurysm or weakening of an arterial wall
    heart failure

SPECIAL CONDITIONS OF YOUR GERIATRIC PATIENT

Determination of heart disease is made by the doctor after physical examination, blood tests, blood pressure readings, and an electrocardiogram (E.K.G.).

ELECTROCARDIOGRAM (E.K.G. OR E.C.G.)

An E.K.G. machine is an electric box (usually mounted on a wheeled table) that has wires attached to it, which are glued to the skin of the patient's chest, arms, and legs. A trained person operates a panel on the box to measure the patient's heart activity and to trace it on graph paper. The tracing is then studied for differences from normal tracings.

ACUTE SYMPTOMS

Patients without previous signs of heart or blood vessel disease sometimes develop acute symptoms, and patients with chronic disease sometimes have acute attacks. Acute symptoms include severe chest pain, difficulty in breathing, blue color to skin, irregular pulse, anxiety, and dizziness. Whenever acute symptoms develop, the patient requires special care. If he is very ill, he may be moved to a hospital or coronary care unit where a cardiac monitor can be used. A coronary care unit is a special area provided with machines and personnel to observe and give intensive care to a heart patient.

CARDIAC MONITOR

A cardiac monitor is an electric machine that can be attached by wire to the patient's skin. The machine records a continuous pattern of the patient's heart activity and shows the activity on a television-like screen. A trained observer can read the patient's immediate condition by a glance at the screen.

CARE OF PATIENTS WITH ACUTE SYMPTOMS

Other aspects of care of patients with acute symptoms may include the following:
rest
positioning
oxygen
special diet
intravenous feedings to regulate the sodium and potassium balance of the blood
medication

REST

Physical Rest

The doctor orders complete bed rest (CBR) at first and then gradual activity.
He orders mild laxatives to keep the patient's bowels open so that there is no danger of an attack through straining to expel a hard stool. Be alert for any sign of constipation and report it at once.
Move the patient as gently as possible. (Passive exercises may be ordered.)
Anticipate the patient's needs so he does not have to speak.
Provide a pleasant, airy, comfortable room with no bright lights.

Keep the room as free of noise as possible.
Be pleasant and cheerful but not talkative.
Give special care to the patient's skin to prevent breakdown.

Mental Rest

At first the patient is not allowed to read, watch television, or listen to the radio.
A telephone should be removed from the room.
He should be assured about business or his concern for his family.

Emotional Rest

Visiting is allowed only as the doctor orders and, at first, is usually restricted to family. Visits should be short, a few minutes at a time, and talking limited. Visitors must be warned not to upset the patient by weeping or telling him about problems.

You must stop the visit at any small sign of distress or fatigue on the part of the patient.

POSITIONING IN BED

The body is placed in a position that makes it easiest for the patient to breath. The patient's head and chest are elevated. Supports, such as pillows, are put under his knees and forearms. Sometimes he is positioned sitting and bent forward in the bed with his arms resting on an overbed table that has been padded with pillows.

If the doctor orders *keep head of bed elevated,* you must not lower it at any time, even to make the bed. In most facilities, when such an order is written, a warning sign is placed at the foot of the bed. (*Example:* Do Not Lower Head of Bed.)

OXYGEN (O$_2$)

(*See* Chap. 15, "Your Geriatric Patient Needs Medication and Inhalation Therapy.")
Be sure all safety rules are carried out.
Be sure the liter reading is correct.
Check the amount in the tank often.
Reorder tanks as needed.
Watch and report the patient's reaction to O$_2$.

SPECIAL DIETS

Follow the doctor's orders exactly. He may order any combination of the following diets: soft, low-salt, low-cholesterol, or low-calorie, as well as other specific diet requirements.

If the patient is in a nursing facility, the diet is prepared by the diet kitchen. If the patient is at home, you can easily prepare his food by using a diet sheet provided by the doctor.

Soft Diet

(*See* Chap. 9, "Your Geriatric Patient Needs Food and Fluid Balance.")

SPECIAL CONDITIONS OF YOUR GERIATRIC PATIENT

Low-Sodium or Low-Salt Diet

Use no salt in cooking or preparing foods.

Use fresh vegetables and fruits.

Do not use any canned or frozen foods unless they are labeled *unsalted* or *salt-free*.

Do not use any packaged mix such as pancake, muffin, or cake.

Remove salt shaker from the tray or table.

Use salt-free butter or margarine.

Do not use corned products such as beef or tongue.

Do not use frankfurters or luncheon meats or salted fish.

Do not use ready-to-eat cereals except Puffed Rice or Puffed Wheat.

Read food labels. The patient cannot have any sugar substitute that contains sodium. He can have saccharin, if the doctor permits.

Be careful to check any diet drinks sweetened with sugar substitutes.

Use no pickles, relishes, jellies, or packaged gelatins and puddings.

Use unsalted bread and crackers.

Use no cheese except unsalted cottage cheese.

If eating in restaurants, the person on a low-sodium diet should limit himself to those foods to which no salt or monosodium glutamate (a seasoning) is added. These include milk, fresh fruit served whole (but not fruit cocktail or fruit salad, as monosodium glutamate is often added to these), boiled eggs, baked potatoes, broiled meats, fish, and chicken (if a special request is made for them to be prepared without salt).

Sample Low-Salt Diet

Breakfast:
> Fresh orange juice
> Hot cereal cooked without salt
> Boiled egg or unsalted cottage cheese
> Toasted unsalted bread
> Unsalted margarine
> Honey
> Tea or coffee with sugar or saccharin and milk or cream

Lunch:
> Chicken breast (boiled or broiled without added salt)
> Fresh squash (cooked without salt)
> Tossed fresh green salad with oil and fresh lemon juice dressing
> Unsalted melba toast or matzo crackers
> Unsalted margarine
> Tea or coffee with sugar or saccharin and milk or cream

Dinner:
> Broiled or baked meat or fish (prepared without added salt)
> Fresh spinach (cooked without salt)
> Baked potato or boiled rice (cooked without salt)
> Salad of lettuce and sliced fresh tomato with oil and vinegar dressing (no added salt)
> Unsalted bread and unsalted margarine
> Fresh sugared strawberries
> Sponge cake (made without salt)
> Whipped cream
> Coffee or tea with sugar or saccharin and milk or cream

Certain vegetables and fruits have a high natural salt content. Sometimes the doctor will order these vegetables and fruits restricted and his orders must be followed.

One of the most common complaints about a low-salt diet is that the food is tasteless. This can be overcome to a certain extent by preparing foods, such as vegetables, by quick-cooking methods, by using lemon juice at the table instead of a salt shaker, and by preparing foods with a variety of textures. (*Example:* Boiled potato, boiled carrots, and a slice of fresh bread have very similar textures. Baked potato, raw carrot strips, and toast have different textures.) Sodium-free salt substitutes are available at health food stores but should be used only with the doctor's permission.

Low-Cholesterol (Animal Fat) Diet

Use only vegetable oils or margarine in food preparation and at the table. Do not use butter.

Limit egg yolk intake. The doctor will indicate how many eggs a week the patient may have. Notice must be taken of eggs used in cooking; these yolks count too. Foods such as sponge cake and mayonnaise prepared with egg yolks should not be served.

Trim all fat from meat and poultry and use cuts of meat that are less fat. (*Example:* Round steak has much less fat marbling than sirloin.) Do not use ready-ground hamburger. Ask the butcher to grind a piece of completely fat-trimmed round steak instead.

Do not use any cheeses except cottage cheese made from skim milk.

Do not use whole milk, cream, or desserts that include whipped cream.

Skim or fat-free milk may be used.

Do not use meat gravies.

Do not use luncheon meats or canned meat spreads.

Do not use bread, cakes, or pies that use whole milk or butter or lard in their preparation. (Read the label.)

Do not use canned or frozen soups or other foods that contain meat, milk, or chicken fats.

Sample Low-Cholesterol Diet

Breakfast:
>   Fresh fruit or juice
>   Hot cereal with skim milk and sugar or saccharin
>   Toast with margarine and jelly
>   Coffee or tea with skim milk or nondairy creamer

Lunch:
>   Broiled fish filet seasoned with margarine
>   Spinach (cooked in plain manner and without cream sauce)
>   Mashed potatoes (Use skim milk and margarine to prepare.)
>   Green salad with oil and vinegar dressing
>   Water roll and margarine
>   Fruit gelatin with nondairy topping (Read the label.)
>   Coffee or tea with nondairy creamer

Dinner:
>   Baked chicken (Remove all skin and fat from chicken before cooking.)
>   Curried rice (A package mix can be used.)
>   French string beans
>   Angel food cake
>   Canned peaches
>   Coffee or tea with nondairy creamer

Between-meal nourishments of fruit juice, fresh fruit, or skim milk can be used.

Low-Calorie Diet

Prepare all vegetables by quick-cooking methods.

Do not season with butter, salt, oil, cream sauces, or gravies.

Roast, broil, or boil all meat, fish, or poultry.

Remove all fat and skin from meat or poultry before preparing.

Restrict use of bread, cereals, and sugar. Use saccharin if the doctor permits.

Do not serve pies, cakes, ice cream, sour cream, whipped cream, cream, whole milk, cheeses (except for skim-milk cottage cheese), fruits canned in heavy syrup, candy, and so forth.

Do not serve beans, corn, spaghetti, or other pastas.

Sample Low-Calorie and Low-Fat Diet

Breakfast:

Half a grapefruit without sugar

4 oz. of skim-milk cottage cheese

One slice protein bread without butter or margarine

Coffee or tea with skim milk or lemon and saccharin

Mid-Morning:

Cup of low-calorie broth

Lunch:

Large tossed salad of greens, tomatoes, cucumbers, green pepper, and similar ingredients. Use low-calorie commercial dressing or, if restricted in use of salt, 1 tablespoon of vegetable salad oil, herbs, and lemon juice

Two pieces of melba toast

A glass of skim milk

Mid-Afternoon:

A small apple

Dinner:

Small serving of broiled lean fish, meat, or poultry

Two large helpings of cooked vegetables such as green beans, squash, celery, tomatoes, cabbage, brussel sprouts, broccoli, spinach, collards, mustard greens, turnip greens, wax beans, asparagus

One small baked potato without margarine, butter, or sour cream

Cole slaw (made without mayonnaise, oil, or cream)

Slice of melon

Tea or coffee with saccharin and skim milk

Bedtime:

A glass of skim milk or a small piece of fruit

CHRONIC SYMPTOMS

Geriatric patients with chronic heart and blood vessel disease may tire easily, be short of breath, or have irregular breathing, coughing, and wheezing. They may have periods of dizziness, swelling of the ankles and legs, and periods of pain in the chest, neck, and left arm. They may be very pale or very red or have bluish lips and fingernails.

CARE OF PATIENTS WITH CHRONIC SYMPTOMS

Most gerontologists agree that patients with chronic heart disease should be as physically active as possible. Walking and mild exercise are desirable. The patient should avoid emotional stress, mental pressures, and overtiring himself.

He may be more comfortable resting in a sitting position than lying in bed. A large, comfortable armchair with footrest should be provided.

Most gerontologists agree that excess weight contributes to heart and blood vessel problems. The patient therefore should have a diet that will keep him thin.

Tight clothing should never be worn.

He should have frequent reevaluations.

He should have the right medication for his condition.

MEDICATIONS USED IN HEART CARE

As an aide, you should know when a patient is receiving the following medications and what you should expect from the patient as a result of their administration.

Diuretics

This medication draws edema or unwanted fluid from the patient's tissues. As a result, the patient may urinate more frequently. Any patient who is taking a diuretic should be on measured intake and output. (*See* Chap. 9, "Your Geriatric Patient Needs Food and Fluid Balance.")

Nitroglycerine

This medicine dilates blood vessels when a tablet is placed under the tongue. The medicine must be used very quickly by certain patients when they feel approaching distress. This drug is always kept within the patient's ready reach; at night it should be placed on a table at bedside and during the day in a handy pocket of the patient's clothing. The tablet container should be placed in the same locations every night and day.

Oxygen

Sometimes a doctor allows a patient to operate an oxygen tank that is kept at his bedside but used only when the patient feels the need for it. An oxygen mask is the usual form of delivery. When oxygen is used in this way, it is your duty to check the tank frequently and to see that safety precautions are observed.

COMMON RESPIRATORY DISEASES OF GERIATRIC PATIENTS

Emphysema — This is a loss of function in the lungs as a result of air pollution, smoking, and aging. Breathing is difficult.

Tuberculosis, or T.B. — This is an infectious disease caused by a specific organism. It responds well to modern medication.

SPECIAL CONDITIONS OF YOUR GERIATRIC PATIENT

Lung cancer — This is a growth in the lung often caused by irritation from cigarette smoking and air pollution.

Any patient with respiratory problems is more apt to get respiratory infections, such as colds, flus, and pneumonias than is the normal person. Preventive care must be taken.

Many patients have deep coughs that produce sputum. Any such patient should always have at hand a clean disposable container, with a cover, into which he can spit. Containers should be changed daily and more often if necessary. Isolation technique should be used when disposing of containers containing infectious material.

Patients with respiratory problems may receive inhalation therapy to stimulate breathing. They may be taught special breathing and coughing techniques. Postural drainage and steam inhalations may be ordered.

They may move slowly because rapid movements increase breathing difficulties. They may pant, wheeze, whistle, and have bluish or pale and moist skin. Chest movements are usually very noticeable. When in bed these patients should always have their heads elevated because breathing is easiest then.

POSTURAL DRAINAGE

The doctor sometimes orders postural drainage for a patient with respiratory disease. The patient is positioned with head and chest lower than his hips so that secretions can drain from the lungs into the patient's mouth and he can spit them out.

Postural drainage can be done in bed with the patient jackknifed over a fully elevated head rest. Or drainage can be done with the patient lying across the bed with head and shoulders lowered over the side. For the patient who is allowed out of bed, the following method is easy and comfortable.

Giving Postural Drainage Using an Upholstered Armchair

YOU NEED

      a large plastic sheet or newspapers
      a disposal bag
      a large disposable container
      tissues
      a low-backed upholstered armchair

YOU DO THIS

Cover the chair seat, arms and seat back with the plastic sheet or newspapers.

Place the disposable container in the center of the chair seat.

Help the patient to stand behind the chair back and to bend over the chair back, so that his elbows rest on the chair arms and his chest and head hang over the container.

Tell him to take deep breaths and to cough so that secretions will loosen and start to drain. Turning from side to side during the coughing and deep breathing helps get drainage from all lung areas.

Have him cover his mouth with tissues while coughing to prevent germ spread.

Place the disposable bag so that the patient can put used tissues in it directly after using them.

As secretions drain tell the patient to spit into the container on the chair seat.

Have the patient remain in drainage position from five to fifteen minutes depending on the doctor's orders and how the patient responds to the treatment.

Watch the patient for signs of weakness, dizziness or overtiring. Stop the treatment if this occurs.

SPUTUM SPECIMEN

Sputum is material coughed up from the lungs. The usual time to collect a sputum specimen is just after a patient has awakened from the night.

Take the bedside sputum cup away from the patient and give him the collection container.

Have the patient cough deeply for several minutes and then spit into the collection container.

Use a sterile disposable tongue depressor or plastic spoon to transfer some of the sputum into a sterile specimen jar.

Do not refrigerate.

21

CARING FOR THE GERIATRIC PATIENT WITH VISION LOSS
AND HEARING LOSS

STUDY GUIDE

Failing Vision

Of what is a geriatric person with poor vision afraid?

Tell eight special safety measures that protect the patient with failing vision.

Tell four special ways to behave with a person who has poor sight.

What visual aids are available for those with poor vision?

Tell how to take care of eyeglasses.

Tell how the belongings of a person with poor sight should be marked.

What five things can a marking tell the person with poor sight?

Tell how to mark a slipover sweater so that the patient can tell the front from the back and the color.

Tell how to keep a pair of gloves together for washing, drying, and storing.

Tell how to arrange the closet of a person with poor vision so that he can identify clothing by placement and touch.

Tell how to arrange the drawers of a person with failing sight.

Tell how to feed a patient with poor vision.

Hearing Loss

What does the person with hearing loss need?

What kinds of hearing aids are available?

Tell how to care for a hearing aid.

Give six ways to behave with a person with hearing loss.

From what does a person with hearing loss need to be protected?

FAILING VISION

Among geriatric patients can be found those who are blind. Most of these, however, are not blind as a result of aging and, therefore, have had special training in adapting to their handicaps. More common among the aged are those with poor or failing vision.

It is necessary only to close your eyes for a few minutes and to attempt to carry on your everyday life in order to experience the confusion that a person with poor vision feels. The geriatric patient feels more. He is afraid of falling or otherwise hurting himself, afraid of being cut off from the normal life of people who can see, and afraid of losing his independence. All of these fears can be calmed.

Special Safety Measures

(*See* Chap. 3, "Your Geriatric Patient Needs a Clean, Safe, Comfortable Place.")
Remove unnecessary furniture from his room.
Remove throw rugs and anything else that can cause the patient to trip.
Do not wax floors.
Arrange the furniture to suit his needs and to provide clear pathways to the bathroom and room exit door. Use a guide rope to these areas if necessary.
Remove fragile glass objects that can shatter.
Have the room well lighted.
Block stairs and other dangerous areas.
If he enters a strange room, describe the room and its contents to him. If he is able, take him around the room so that he could touch the contents and orient himself.
Never leave a person with poor vision on the direct path of an obstacle. (*Example:* Never leave a patient facing a wheelchair or a wall.)
When helping the person to a seat, put his hand on the arm or back of the chair. If this is impossible, walk up to the chair with him so that he is facing it. Tell him the location of the chair.
See that the person dresses in neat, becoming clothes, that his hair is trimmed and combed, and that his whiskers are shaved. Encourage a woman to use makeup and wear jewelry.

Special Social Manners

See that the person with failing vision is included in groups that watch television or movies, plays, and sporting events. He is as interested in life and social contact as is a person who sees well.
Always address a blind person or one with failing vision directly, by name, and not through another person. (*Example:* Don't say, "Does he take tea or coffee?" Say, "Will you have coffee or tea, Mr. Smith?")
Always identify yourself before talking to the person with poor vision. Unless he knows you extremely well, he cannot identify you by your voice. (*Example:* Say, "It's Miss Jones, Mr. Smith. I've brought your breakfast.")
Always let the person know when you are leaving him so that he doesn't continue talking after you have gone. (*Example:* Say, "I have to leave you now, Mr. Jones.")
When walking with a person who has poor vision, let him take your arm rather than your taking his. He can better balance himself and sense your moves if he holds onto you. If the way is too narrow to walk arm in arm, you go first, extending your arm behind you to take hold of his hand. While you walk single file, talk to him, describing anything in the way so that he is prepared for your movements. (*Example:* Say, "There's a table in our way just ahead. I'm going to move left to go around it.")

SPECIAL CONDITIONS OF YOUR GERIATRIC PATIENT

Visual Aids

Most geriatric patients wear eyeglasses and are very dependent on them. In addition to eyeglasses, they may use hand-held or stand magnifying glasses. Large-print books and newspapers are available.

Care of Eyeglasses

Check eyeglasses daily. They should be free of smudges, dust, and spots on the lenses. If you are cleaning lenses with a special eyeglass cleaning product, read the instructions on the label and follow them. Know if the lenses are glass or plastic. Never use polishing paper on plastic lenses.

The eyeglasses should sit straight and snug on the bridge of the nose. If hinges or earpieces are loose, the glasses can slip forward or be seated crooked, distorting vision. If earpieces are very loose, glasses may fall off when the patient looks down.

The glasses should not pinch, put pressure on, rub, or redden any part of the patient's nose or ears. If any of these things occurs, the glasses should be adjusted by a specialist and skin care given to the affected area.

Eyeglasses should always be stored in a protective pouch to prevent scratching or breaking. Never lay eyeglasses lens down on a hard surface.

Eyeglasses should always be kept in the same safe place within the patient's easy reach.

They should never be worn by anyone except the person to whom they were fitted.

Marking Belongings

The belongings of a geriatric person with failing vision, but who is otherwise able, should be marked so that he can identify them by touch. This allows the patient to perform a maximum of self-care. A simple marking system can be taught to the patient and the patient encouraged to help in doing the marking. The patient should be able to identify the following:

> which items belong to him
> one item from another
> the front from the back of a garment
> one color from another
> two of a pair, such as gloves or socks

When a patient must share storage space, such as a medicine cabinet, his toilet items can be identified if a rubber band or adhesive tape strip is put around each.

Different-sized containers help him to identify one product from another. Color markings help him to tell one garment from another.

Sew-on or iron-on tape in the center back of collars and waistbands allows him to tell front from back.

Sewing thread knots on the tape can be used to identify color. (*Example:* One knot for blue, and two knots for brown.)

Shoes can be marked for color by putting tape strips on the underarch. (*Example:* One strip for blue, and two strips for brown.)

When numbers of knots and tapes are used for colors, the same number should stand for the same color, regardless of marking material. (*Example:* One should always be blue and two always brown, regardless of whether the marking material is tape or knots.)

Two socks or gloves can easily be kept mated if the two of a pair are pinned together with a safety pin when the patient removes them. They can be washed, dried, and stored while pinned, and unpinned only when the patient is wearing them. (Use brass safety pins to prevent rusting.)

Arranging Closets

Hang all clothing of one kind together and always in the same place. (*Example:* Hang all long coats on the far right of a closet and all jackets on the near right.)

Hang clothing according to frequency of use. For example, the everyday coat should be first in the coat group, with raincoat next, and dress coat last.

If plastic clothing bags are used, mark each, in the same place near the zipper pull, with short strips of plastic tape to indicate the contents of the bag. (*Example:* One strip for dresses, two strips for coats, and three strips for slacks.)

Keep shoes together in pairs in boxes or a door shoebag. Boxes can be marked with plastic tape strips to identify the shoes. (*Example:* One strip for high heels, and two strips for low heels.) If a bag is used, keep pairs together in rows. (*Example:* First row, low heels; second row, high heels.)

Arranging Drawers

Use boxes without covers as drawer dividers, and put all items of a kind into one box. For example, in all average dresser drawers, two shirt laundry boxes can provide three space divisions. Put shirts with front openings in one box, collarless slipover shirts in the other box, and turtleneck shirts in the space between them.

In shallow drawers, plastic egg cartons make good dividers for small objects.

Feeding the Patient

Unless the patient is too ill to do so, he should feed himself. He can manage very well if you do the following:

Protect his clothing with a bib or napkin.

Be sure he is in a comfortable eating position and that his tray or table setting is easy to reach.

Set his tray with as few dishes and as little equipment as possible.

Describe to him the location of every article on the tray and exactly what food or drink each dish or cup contains.

When describing a plate containing several kinds of food, have the patient imagine the plate to be the face of a clock. Then, describe the food in relationship to the clock. Say, "You have sliced carrots at eleven o'clock, mashed potatoes at three o'clock, and chopped steak at six o'clock." Meat is always positioned at six o'clock. With this image, the blind person has no difficulty in locating and selecting what he chooses to eat.

Prepare his food before he begins. Put sugar and milk on his cereal if he wants them. Butter his bread and cut his meat if he cannot manage otherwise.

Let him taste the food, then ask if he would like additional salt or pepper, and so forth.

Have cups or glasses only three-quarters full. Use plasticware rather than china or glass.

Put straws in liquids.

Do not serve liquids that are very hot. Warn him of hot dishes or foods.

Try to avoid serving foods that are difficult for even the sighted to eat, such as peas, or prepare them in such a way as to make them manageable. (*Example:* Serve peas as pea soup or mix the peas with mashed potatoes.)

If you must feed the patient, sit down beside him. Relax and make pleasant conversation or he will sense your rush and become nervous. Offer small bites. Tell the patient which food is in each bite, whether the bite is on a fork or a spoon, and whether that bite is hot or cold. If he is very ill or deaf, touch his cheek to signal that the spoon is ready.

(HEARING LOSS)

Although some geriatric people retain adequate hearing throughout their lives, most develop some dysfunction that interferes with communication. The person with hearing loss needs adaptive equipment or other aids to communication; he needs to be included in the social life of others, and he needs special efforts on the part of others to communicate with him.

Hearing Aids

Many patients can be helped with hearing aids. Some of these are so small that they can be fitted into the earpiece of eyeglasses or worn as an earring to button in the ear canal. Earpieces for radio and television listening allow some who need amplified hearing to listen without disturbing others.

Care of Hearing Aids

Check the aid daily for proper function.
Clean the earpiece with a moist, but not wet, alcohol sponge.
Store the aid within the patient's easy reach.
Store the aid in a protected place where it cannot fall or otherwise be damaged.
Report any change in the aid or the patient's ability to use it to the charge nurse.

Special Social Manners

Always face the person and look directly at him, regardless of whether you or he is speaking.
Don't make noises, such as shuffling your feet, coughing, or clapping your hands, when conversing with him.
Keep room background noises to a minimum. (*Example:* Close a window on a noisy street or turn off a television before conversing with the person.)
Listen to him attentively. Many people with hearing loss also suffer some speech difficulty.
Never shout, but do speak slowly and distinctly.
If he has a hearing aid, see that he uses it during conversation.
See that he always has within his easy reach a pad and pencil so that he can write or read if he fails to communicate through speech or hearing.

Special Protection

Hearing can be affected by head colds, wind, and dust. The person with hearing loss should be protected from these.

22

CARING FOR THE GERIATRIC FRACTURE PATIENT

STUDY GUIDE

What is the best geriatric fracture care?

When a fracture occurs in an older patient, how may it otherwise affect the patient?

What routine nursing care should a geriatric fracture patient receive in addition to special care?

Tell what you need to give first aid to a fracture patient.

Tell how to give first aid to a fracture patient.

How does a doctor treat a fracture?

How is a cast applied?

Tell how to care for a patient with a cast.

What is traction?

Tell four ways in which traction can be applied.

Tell how to care for a patient in weight traction.

AGING makes people more accident prone. Diseases waste the body. Muscles lose tone. Eyesight, hearing, and touch sensitivity become less acute and lessen the person's ability to recognize danger. Slower reflexes reduce the ability to withdraw from danger. Mental confusion often interferes with an understanding of danger. Older people bump against objects, trip, slip, and fall more frequently than do younger adults. Since bones tend to grow brittle with age, a hard bump or a minor fall can cause a fracture.

The best geriatric fracture care, therefore, is preventive. All older people should be protected against the possibility of injury. Safety devices and techniques should be used in every aspect of geriatric care. (*See* Chap. 3, "Your Geriatric Patient Needs a Clean, Safe, Comfortable Place.")

When a fracture does occur, the older patient does not heal quickly, and shock from the injury can disturb health in many dangerous ways. Mental confusion, digestive upset, incontinence, bowel impaction, skin breakdown, pneumonia, pain, and stiffness are frequent complications of fractures in geriatric patients.

Every effort must be made to prevent these conditions and to treat any accident or complication immediately. You must observe the fracture patient with special care, report and discuss with the charge nurse or doctor any changes in the patient's condition, and give emotional support as well as physical attention. In addition to other special nursing care, a geriatric fracture patient should receive the following as a routine:

>intensive skin care
>
>changing position every 2 hours (q.2.h.)
>
>careful supervision of fluid and food intake
>
>careful bowel and bladder control

KINDS OF FRACTURE

A simple fracture is a break in the bone, but the bone does not pierce the skin.

A compound fracture is a break in a bone and the bone does pierce the skin.

FIRST AID

First aid for a fracture involves treatment for shock and application of a splint to the affected body part. No effort should be made to undress, manipulate, or to otherwise adjust the fractured part. The splint helps prevent movement in the broken part until the patient can be treated by a doctor.

Bleeding can be controlled by a pressure bandage to the open area.

Giving First Aid

YOU NEED

blankets or other warm coverings

4 or more strong cloth strips

a splint: any firm, straight, lightweight object that is about the length of the broken part

padding for the broken part

YOU DO THIS

Reassure the patient.

Leave the patient where he has fallen or help him to lie down.

Place the patient in the supine position. Use care in extending the broken part.

Loosen any tight clothing.

SPECIAL CONDITIONS OF YOUR GERIATRIC PATIENT

Use the blankets to cover all the patient's body except the affected part.

Put padding around the part.

Lay the splint beside the part so that the fracture is in the center of the splint.

Without tying, gently arrange all the cloth strips in position around the affected part and the splint so that the ends of the ties are on the outside of the splint.

Keeping the tension steady but not overly tight, knot the ties securely, tying them in the order of placement, and positioning the knots against the splint.

Commercial plastic inflatable splints are available in a variety of sizes. Such splints offer excellent, lightweight protection for emergency care and should be part of the standard equipment of any geriatric facility.

TREATMENT OF A FRACTURE

A doctor treats a fracture by *reduction*. This means that he pulls and adjusts bone edges until they are in normal position.

If the break is simple, the doctor may do a *closed reduction,* or one that does not require surgery. If the break is compound, the doctor may do an *open reduction,* or one that requires surgery.

Sometimes a doctor performs surgery on either a simple or a compound fracture in order to insert a metal pin, nail, plate, or screw into the bone to brace the break. This is called *internal fixation*. It is often used on geriatric patients because it allows more body motion than an external cast and, therefore, helps prevent health complications.

After reduction of the fracture, the doctor maintains correct positioning by applying a cast or traction to the broken part.

A *cast* is a hard covering molded to fit a body part so that the part maintains a fixed position. *Traction* is the use of pulling force to correct and maintain normal positioning.

APPLICATION OF A CAST

After reducing a fracture, the doctor covers all the body part to be contained by the cast with soft cotton stockinette. He then wets plaster gauze and applies it over the stockinette to build a thick shell. This hardens as it dries and braces and protects the break during healing.

CARE OF A PATIENT WITH A CAST

A cast takes a long time to dry and may still be damp when the patient is put to bed.

YOU DO THIS

Use a bedboard to make the mattress firm.

Protect bedding by using a plastic mattress cover or a plastic drawsheet under the cast area.

Use only the palms of your hands to handle a damp cast. Fingers can cause pressure indentations in the cast.

Use small pillows under the curves of the cast to prevent the cast from cracking or changing shape.

Cover all the body except that in the cast with a sheet or bath blanket. Leave the cast exposed to dry.

Turn the patient often to ensure even drying of the cast and to prevent skin pressure points.

Cover the parts of the cast that may be soiled by urine or feces with disposable plastic-backed padding.

Watch the skin around the cast and fingers or toes for changes in color to very white or blue.

Also watch for swelling. Report such signs to the head nurse or doctor at once.

Also report at once if the patient complains of numbness, pain, or tingling in the area covered by the cast.

An arm or a leg in a cast should be elevated to lessen swelling.

After the cast is dry, use self-adhering foam padding that is cut to size to pad pressure points made by the cast.

TRACTION

Traction is the use of sustained pulling force to correct and maintain body positioning. Traction can be applied in several ways:

        by weights
        by elastic
        by special clothing
        by skeletal bracing

Weight traction is applied by attaching one end of a rope to the extremity of the affected body part and stringing the other end over a pulley and weighting it. The poundage of the weights for each traction is specified by the doctor. Only people with special training can apply weight traction.

In *elastic traction*, an elastic appliance causes pull on the affected part.

Special clothing that braces and limits movement is usually made of combinations of leather, metal, plastic, and strong cloth. Surgical collars and corsets are examples of special traction clothing.

In *skeletal traction*, a doctor performs surgery to attach pins, wires, or tongs directly onto the bone.

Care of the Patient in Weight Traction

Special skin care is necessary to prevent skin breakdown at pressure areas.

The patient's position must be changed on a regular schedule.

The doctor may order an overhead trapeze so that the patient can use it to lift himself when changing position. The patient should be taught and frequently reminded to pull straight on the bar when lifting himself. By doing so, he does not disturb the traction.

Both the patient and the traction equipment should be checked by all nursing personnel whenever they are approaching the bed.

See that traction weights always hang free. (They should never be allowed to rest on a chair, the floor, or part of the bed.)

See that the patient has not slipped down in the bed. If he has, reposition him.

See that the patient is positioned so that nothing interferes with the traction.

When making the bed of a patient in traction, start making it on the patient's affected side. This disturbs the traction less.

If the patient complains of feeling chilled or if the affected part feels cold to your touch, cover the part in traction with a baby blanket or other lightweight covering.

23

CARING FOR THE GERIATRIC PATIENT WHO IS DYING

STUDY GUIDE

How have attitudes about death and dying changed?

What five emotional stages does a dying person experience?

How do geriatric patients accept death?

What right has become important to older patients?

How may the dying patient appear?

What happens to the sensory awareness of a dying patient?

How does your staying with the patient help him?

Should you talk about the patient's condition so that he can hear you?

How can you help family and friends of the patient?

Tell some special ways in which you should treat the dying patient.

What changes may occur in the skin, pulse, and respiration just before death?

What should you do when the patient stops breathing?

Who pronounces the patient dead?

What type of notes should be made on the chart of a person after his death?

What attentions must be given to a body soon after death?

Tell what you need to give postmortem care.

Tell how to give postmortem care.

DEATH AND DYING

Not so long ago, few patients were allowed to discuss dying and death. Doctors, nursing personnel, and families conspired to hide from patients the deadly possibilities of illness. However, in recent years, researchers have studied the psychological effects that dying and death have upon patients and their families. These researchers have found that except in sudden death, a dying person usually goes through five progressive emotional stages other than fear and anxiety.

When confronted with death, a person's first reaction is denial. It is very difficult for one to imagine his own death. Death seems to be something that happens to others. A person thinks, "It can't happen to me!"

After he realizes that he can die, his second reaction is anger. He feels singled out for misery. He asks, "Why me?" And then he defies death. He says, "I won't die!"

When death continues to threaten, the person enters a third stage. He begins to bargain for his life. He says such things as, "I'm going to give up all my bad habits if I get well!" Or he might say, "If I get out of this, I'm going to give all my money to benefit others."

But as the dying process goes on, the patient has a fourth reaction. He becomes very depressed. At first, the depression is a form of grief because he must leave life. The patient may cry, withdraw from the attentions of family and friends or even become hostile to them. He may refuse food, be unable to sleep and feel sorry for himself. Later, his thinking shifts from looking back on life to looking forward to death. He may appear to be more cooperative but actually be more withdrawn. He may say little, sigh often, and stare into space.

In time he reaches the last stage, which is one of acceptance. Depression leaves him and he becomes calm about his fate, awaiting death with patience and dignity.

One important result of these studies has been the discovery that many patients want to talk about dying, want to express their feelings, and want to plan the rest of their lives. Talking and expressing feelings help them through the four stages that precede acceptance of death. And talking may help the family to adjust their lives to the loss.

Geriatric patients usually accept death more willingly than younger adults. Death may even seem attractive to those who have lost many family members and friends; whose life style has been changed by disability, pain, and limited income. Many older people have been threatened by death several times and so have experienced the five emotional stages of dying. Some have more fear of continued life than of dying.

In fact, the right to die has become an important issue among older people. Legal forms are now available for patients to sign. These forms request that in the event of extreme conditions, no special efforts be made to prolong the signer's life.

Your duties, when working with older patients who are dying, are to observe and report signs of emotional changes as well as physical symptoms, to discuss such changes with the charge nurse or doctor, to listen to patients who express their feelings and to give them whatever emotional support and physical attentions they may need.

The dying patient is often in physical distress and frightened. He may be extremely restless, gasping for breath, and disoriented. He may appear comatose or unconscious.

Even when he appears to be disoriented or unconscious, he may in fact have increased awareness of light, sounds, movements near him, touch, smell, and other sensory stimulants.

Every effort must be made to reduce irritating conditions and provide a comfortable, reassuring situation.

YOU DO THIS

Comfort the patient by staying with him as much as possible. Be very careful of conversation with the patient, visitors, and personnel and of their conversation with each other. Do not say anything that can cause the patient mental distress.

Relieve suffering with your most conscientious nursing care.

See that the patient has the comfort of his religion.

Be sympathetic with family and friends. Protect them from sights and sounds that would cause them distress.

Keep the room light and aired. Try to prevent any objectionable odors by keeping the patient as clean as possible.

Keep the patient warm, but make the top bedding light in weight and tuck it over a footboard to free the feet.

Give special mouth care, every hour, to keep the mouth moist. A thin application of oil over the lips prevents dryness.

Handle the patient very gently but change his position often. Placing the patient on his side helps mucus drain from the mouth or nose.

Check urinary output and be sure the patient does not have a full bladder to distress him. The doctor may order a catheterization if the bladder is full.

Check the skin color, respirations, and pulse frequently. Mark them down. Report any changes to the charge nurse. Just before death the skin may become cold and damp, the respirations long, drawn out, and interrupted, the pulse very irregular.

When the patient stops breathing, take notice of the exact time. Check the pulse. Call the charge nurse or doctor. A doctor must be summoned to pronounce the person dead.

Escort family or friends from the room and to a private area where they can express their grief without disturbing other patients.

Give the charge nurse your notes on pulse, respiration, skin color, any changes in the patient's behavior, visits by any doctors, the exact time that respiration ceased, the name of the doctor who pronounced the patient dead, and the time at which he died. All this information must be charted.

GIVING POSTMORTEM OR AFTER-DEATH CARE

Certain necessary attentions must be given a body soon after death to keep it as natural-looking as possible. These are done in any situation, because the body stiffens as heat leaves it. Once hardened, body parts do not move.

The body is laid flat on the back with one pillow under the head.
The eyes are closed.
Any dentures or other artificial parts, such as an eye, are placed in position on the body.
The body is cleaned.
The hands are folded on the chest.

The body and the possessions must be plainly identified in a hospital or nursing home. At home the undertaker identifies and gives all further care to the body.

In many nursing homes, an undertaker gives all further care.

General Hospital or Nursing Home Procedure

YOU NEED

T-binder or triangular bandage

cotton pads

safety pins

padding and wrapping for the hands and feet

padding and wrapping for the jaw

3 identification tags

a shroud or sheet

equipment for bathing the body

dressings and adhesive tape for wounds

remover for taking off adhesive marks

YOU DO THIS

Draw the unit curtains closed.

Lower the bed so that it is flat.

Arrange the body flat on its back with one pillow under the head.

Close the eyes. If the eyes are not closed very soon after death, it is difficult to close them.

Replace false teeth and other prostheses.

Remove any jewelry except for a wedding ring.

Remove any drainage tubes.

Remove any dressings. Close wounds with adhesive.

Remove old adhesive marks with remover.

Bathe the body. Comb the hair.

Pad and wrap the jaw. Padding is important to prevent pressure marks. The jaw is wrapped because it has a tendency to fall open.

SPECIAL CONDITIONS OF YOUR GERIATRIC PATIENT

Pad and wrap the urinary and anal areas. The muscles that control these areas relax at death and release the bladder and bowel contents.

Pad and tie the wrists together on the chest. This places them in the position in which they will be in the coffin.

Pad and tie the ankles together. This keeps the legs straight and together.

Fill out three identification tags and tie one to a wrist. The body goes to the hospital morgue, and from there, it is taken by an undertaker. Identification is necessary.

Put the shroud on the body.

Tie an identification tag to the outside of the shroud.

Check and list every item of the patient's belongings.

Bundle all of the patient's belongings together and attach the third identification card to the bundle.

Give the bundle to the head nurse. She sees that the family or proper receiver takes them.

Draw the curtains of any other patients in the same room. This is so they will not be alarmed by the sight of the body being removed.

Ask all ambulatory patients to return to their beds.

Close all the doors in the hallway.

Get a stretcher and someone to help you.

Return to the bedside. Lift the body onto the stretcher. Cover and secure it.

Take the body to the freight elevator, or ring and notify the elevator operator so that he can empty his car of passengers before wheeling the stretcher to the elevator.

Take the body to the morgue and give it to the morgue attendant.

Remember to always handle the body with respect.

Return to the ward.

Open closed doors and drawn screens, except around the deceased or dead person's unit.

Clean and care for all equipment and the unit.

SAMPLE EXAMINATIONS

Examination 1

There is one correct statement in each group of three sentences. Put a check beside each correct statement.

A. ( ) A urinary catheter is always inserted under sterile conditions.
    ( ) An aide can insert a urinary catheter.
    ( ) A urinary catheter is inserted to relieve flatus.
B. ( ) A geriatric patient should do as little for himself as possible.
    ( ) A geriatric patient should do as much for himself as he is able.
    ( ) A geriatric patient should never do anything for himself.
C. ( ) Geriatric patients do not need side rails on their beds.
    ( ) Side rails need not be raised at night.
    ( ) Side rails should always be raised on the beds of confused patients.
D. ( ) A depressed patient should be kept away from other patients.
    ( ) A depressed patient should be left alone in his room until he feels better.
    ( ) A depressed patient should have social contact and be encouraged to talk with others.

Examination 2

Some of the following statements are true and some are false. Write the word *yes* next to all statements that are true. Write the word *no* next to all statements that are false.

1. Only incontinent patients need skin care. _____
2. Any piece of walking equipment should be examined before and after use for wear. _____
3. Skin care should be given to areas subjected to pressure by a brace. _____
4. Geriatric patients should do range of motion exercises for an hour once a day. _____
5. A helpless bed patient should be turned every two hours during both day and night or on all three work shifts. _____
6. The temperature of bath water for a geriatric patient should be 125°F. _____
7. A patient on a bowel retraining program should be scolded if he is incontinent. _____
8. A patient with an A.D.L. eating device should be encouraged to feed himself although he may take longer to do so. _____

323

9. Every geriatric patient should have a hot bath every morning. _____
10. A doctor or podiatrist should trim the toenails of a diabetic patient. _____

Examination 3

Find the correct definition for each of the terms in the left column and write the number of the correct definition in the second column.

A.D.L.	_____	1. Patient record card
Podiatrist	_____	2. Nursing home patient
Cardex	_____	3. Movable toilet chair
P.T.	_____	4. Activities of daily living
O.T.	_____	5. Doctor who specializes in care of the aged
Geriatrician	_____	6. Physical therapy
Resident	_____	7. Foot specialist
Commode	_____	8. Range of motion exercises
R.O.M.	_____	9. A mechanical respirator
Bird	_____	10. Occupational therapy

SAMPLE EXAMINATIONS

CORRECT ANSWERS

Examination 1

A. A urinary catheter is always inserted under sterile conditions.
B. A geriatric patient should do as much for himself as he is able.
C. Side rails should always be raised on the beds of confused patients.
D. A depressed patient should have social contact and be encouraged to talk with others.

Examination 2

1. No
2. Yes
3. Yes
4. No
5. Yes
6. No
7. No
8. Yes
9. No
10. Yes

Examination 3

A.D.L.	_____	4
Podiatrist	_____	7
Cardex	_____	1
P.T.	_____	6
O.T.	_____	10
Geriatrician	_____	5
Resident	_____	2
Commode	_____	3
R.O.M.	_____	8
Bird	_____	9

Index

STUDENT WORK RECORD

Name   Class   Starting Date

Circle each announced lecture number that you attend: 1 2 3 4 5 6 7 8 9 10 11 12 13 14 15 16

17 18 19 20 21 22 23 24 25 26 27 28 29 30

DEMONSTRATION RECORD

Program 1	Date Observed	Date Practiced	Date Practiced	Teacher's Approval
1.				
2.				
3.				
4.				
5.				
6.				
7.				
8.				
9.				
10.				
11.				
12.				

Program 2				
1.				
2.				
3.				
4.				
5.				
6.				
7.				
8.				
9.				
10.				
11.				
12.				

Program 3				
1.				
2.				
3.				
4.				
5.				
6.				
7.				
8.				
9.				
10.				
11.				
12.				